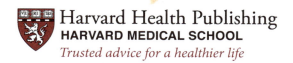

Dear Reader,

The total number of Americans with high blood pressure rose sharply in late 2017—but not because people suddenly became less healthy. Instead, new guidelines from the American Heart Association and the American College of Cardiology lowered the threshold for diagnosing this common condition, which is known medically as hypertension. Before the update, high blood pressure was defined as a reading of 140/90 millimeters of mercury (mm Hg) or higher. Now, anyone with a reading of 130/80 mm Hg or above is considered to have high blood pressure. Nearly half of American adults—about 46%—fall into this group. If you are among the millions of Americans who suddenly qualified as having high blood pressure, it may be tempting to ignore the new findings. But the updated guidelines are based on a growing body of evidence showing that lower blood pressure values are associated with fewer heart attacks and strokes.

High blood pressure has no symptoms or warning signs. Yet it can be so dangerous to your health and well-being, it has earned the nickname "the silent killer." Over all, people with Stage 1 hypertension—people who didn't even qualify as having hypertension before the new guidelines came out—have double the risk of heart attacks and strokes as people with normal blood pressure. If you have elevated pressure along with abnormal cholesterol and blood sugar levels, or if you also smoke, the damage to your arteries, kidneys, and heart accelerates exponentially.

Fortunately, high blood pressure is easy to detect and treat. In some cases, you can bring blood pressure into a normal range without medication, simply by adopting basic lifestyle changes—such as eating more fruits and vegetables, exercising more, and practicing stress reduction techniques. In terms of healthy eating, there's a clear mandate to eat less salt, the primary source of sodium in the diet. The Special Section in this report details numerous strategies you can use to conquer your salt habit on your own.

In this report, you'll also find information about other dietary changes that can help you lose weight and lower your blood pressure, tips on using home blood pressure monitors, and a detailed explanation of blood pressure medications and how they work. More than 200 medications are available to control hypertension. That means if one drug doesn't work or causes unwanted side effects, chances are good that another one will work for you. By working with your health care providers and following the advice in this report, you can disarm the silent killer—and lead a much healthier life.

Sincerely,

Randall M. Zusman, M.D.
Medical Editor

Blood pressure basics

You can't see your blood pressure or feel it, so you may wonder why this simple measure of health is so important. The answer is that your blood pressure gives your doctor a peek into the workings of your circulatory system. A high number means that your heart is working harder to pump blood through your body. This extra work can result in a thickened heart muscle and potential heart, kidney, and brain damage down the road. Your arteries also suffer when your blood pressure is high. The relentless pounding of the blood against the artery walls causes an accumulation of cholesterol deposits, which can diminish blood flow and potentially set you up for a heart attack, stroke, or kidney failure.

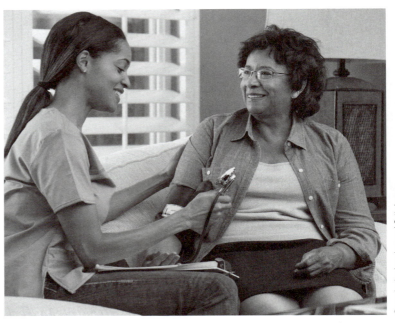

Taking your blood pressure gives your doctor a peek into your circulatory system. The higher the reading, the harder your heart is working.

Having your blood pressure measured is a familiar ritual at most visits to the doctor's office. The examiner inflates a cuff around your upper arm, listens through a stethoscope, watches a gauge while deflating the cuff, and then scribbles some numbers on your chart. Be sure to ask what the reading is each time, because health care professionals don't always tell you. When you find out, make sure to keep a record of this information. Readings can fluctuate, and the more of them you have, the truer picture you will get of how high your blood pressure actually is. But what do these numbers mean?

Understanding the numbers

Blood pressure is recorded as millimeters of mercury (mm Hg) because the traditional measuring device, called a sphygmomanometer, uses a glass column that's filled with mercury and is marked in millimeters. A rubber tube connects the column to an arm cuff. As the cuff is inflated or deflated, mercury rises and falls within the column (see Figure 1, page 3). Although mercury gauges are still considered the gold standard for measuring blood pressure, mercury-free devices are available. Many modern instruments use a spring gauge with a round dial or a digital monitor, but even these are calibrated to give readings in millimeters of mercury.

The top number, or systolic pressure, reflects the amount of pressure during the heart's pumping phase, or systole. As the heart contracts with each beat, pressure in the arteries temporarily increases as blood is forced through them. The bottom number, or diastolic pressure, represents the pressure during the resting phase between heartbeats, or diastole. High blood pressure, also known as hypertension, is defined as having a systolic reading of at least 130 mm Hg or a diastolic reading of at least 80 mm Hg, or both.

To determine whether you have high blood pressure—and if so, how severe it is—a health professional averages two or more readings taken after you have been seated quietly for at least five minutes. For example, a person with a measurement of 125/85 mm Hg on one occasion and 135/95 mm Hg on another has an average blood pressure of 130/90 mm Hg and is said to have Stage 1 hypertension (see Table 1, page 4).

If your blood pressure is above normal, you will most likely need some combination of diet, exercise, stress reduction, and medication to bring it down. Regardless of your blood pressure classification, lifestyle changes should always be the foundation of your treatment. Following is a brief summary of the strategies to consider, depending on which category you fall into.

If your reading is normal

If your blood pressure is below 120/80 mm Hg, this is where you want it to stay. If you are already committed to a healthy lifestyle, keep it up. If you've managed to keep within the normal range without much thought about your health habits, you might want to think again. Even if your blood pressure is normal at age 55, you run a 90% risk of developing high blood pressure within your lifetime. But a combination of exercise, weight loss if needed, limited salt intake, a diet rich in fruits and vegetables, and limits on alcohol consumption can prevent this from happening.

Elevated blood pressure

You have elevated blood pressure if your systolic blood pressure reading is 120 to 129 and your diastolic pressure is less than 80. The risk of cardiovascular disease begins climbing at pressures as low as 115/75 mm Hg, and it doubles for every 20-point increase in systolic pressure and each 10-point increase in diastolic pressure. If your blood pressure falls into the elevated category and you do not have any other risk factors, lifestyle changes are the recommended treatment.

Stage 1 hypertension

You have Stage 1 hypertension if your systolic blood pressure is 130 to 139, your diastolic pressure is 80 to 89, or both. If you don't have any accompanying conditions such as heart disease, diabetes, kidney disease, or a history of stroke, you will usually start with lifestyle modifications and a single medication. Your doctor may let you try lifestyle modifications alone for two or three months to see if you may be

---

Figure 1: Measuring blood pressure

① A clinician wraps a cuff around a person's arm, uses a bulb to inflate the cuff, and listens to the sounds in the brachial (inner arm) artery using a stethoscope.

② When the pressure inside the cuff is greater than the pressure the heart exerts when it contracts (systolic pressure), the cuff squeezes the brachial artery shut. Blood flow stops, so no sounds are heard through the stethoscope.

③ As air is released from the cuff, blood flow resumes through the artery in starts and stops, creating a thumping sound. At that moment, the clinician records the systolic blood pressure.

④ Once the cuff pressure drops below the pressure during the resting phase between heartbeats (diastolic pressure), the thumping sound disappears and the diastolic reading is recorded.

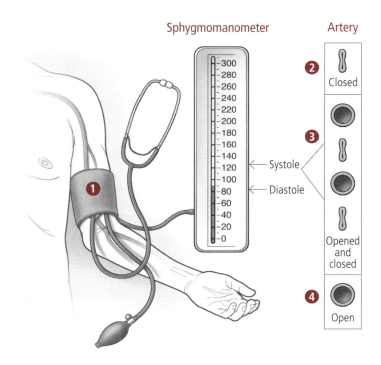

Table 1: Classifying and treating high blood pressure

CATEGORY	SYSTOLIC BLOOD PRESSURE (first number)		DIASTOLIC BLOOD PRESSURE (second number)	WHAT YOU SHOULD DO
Normal	Less than 120	and	Less than 80	Stick with a healthy lifestyle, including following a diet rich in fruits and vegetables and low in sodium, using alcohol moderately, and maintaining a healthy weight.
Elevated	120–129	and	Less than 80	Change health habits. Lose weight if you're overweight. Reduce salt in your diet. Eat more fruits and vegetables, and get more exercise. Drink alcohol only in moderation. You do not need medication at this stage if you don't have other health conditions.
Stage 1 hypertension	130–139	or	80–89	Change your health habits. If you do not have heart disease and are unlikely to develop it in the next decade, you may not need medications.* If your risk is 10% or higher, medication is recommended.
Stage 2 hypertension	140 or higher	or	90 or higher	Change your health habits and take medication. Most people start with one medication, but may need to go to a second or third (or more) to find a treatment that works.
Hypertensive crisis	Higher than 180	and/or	Higher than 120	Consult your doctor immediately.

*People with Stage 1 who have a low (less than 10%) risk of developing heart disease over the next 10 years may not need blood pressure medication, whereas those with a higher risk should consider taking medication. To estimate your risk, use this online calculator: www.cvriskcalculator.com. To use it, you will need to know your total and HDL cholesterol values in addition to your blood pressure reading.

Source: American College of Cardiology and American Heart Association, 2017 Guideline for the Prevention, Detection, Evaluation, and Management of High Blood Pressure in Adults.

able to avoid medication altogether, but many people find that they need to take some type of medication in order to reduce their blood pressure numbers to healthy levels. You may have to try several drugs to find an approach that works well.

The initial choice of drug may depend on whether you have other health problems—such as diabetes, migraine headaches, or cardiac arrhythmias—in addition to hypertension. That's because certain drugs may treat both problems (for example, beta blockers may reduce migraine frequency in addition to lowering blood pressure).

Stage 2 hypertension

You have Stage 2 hypertension if your systolic pressure is at least 140 mm Hg, your diastolic pressure is at least 90 mm Hg, or both. In addition to lifestyle modifications, you will probably need to take at least two medications. If this course of action fails to bring your blood pressure down to your target level (below 130/80 for most individuals, including people with diabetes or chronic kidney disease), your doctor may add additional drugs to the mix.

Regardless of your blood pressure classification, however, lifestyle changes should always be the foundation of your treatment.

How blood pressure changes

Blood pressure reflects both how hard your heart is working and what condition your arteries are in. During strenuous activity, your heart must pump considerably more blood to meet your body's increased demand for oxygen. As blood pushes into the arteries with each heartbeat, it forces the artery walls to expand, much like an elastic waistband stretches to accommodate your body. When the blood flow ebbs, the vessel returns to its original shape. The less flexible the vessels are, the harder it is to propel blood through them—and the higher your blood pressure. Vessels that are narrowed, tightened, or inflexible as a result of plaque buildup over the years have a higher pressure at any level of flow.

Natural blood pressure controls

Your blood pressure is not constant, nor should it be. It fluctuates throughout the day, with lots of small ups and downs punctuated by occasional peaks and valleys. It's generally lowest at night during sleep, when you are placing few demands on your body, and highest in the morning, when you need to rouse your body from sleep and start a new day. It's also higher during exercise, when you need to pump more blood and nutrients to your muscles.

Your body can make dramatic adjustments in blood pressure within seconds to meet sudden demands. A sprint for the elevator or the sound of breaking glass may send blood pressure soaring from an idling 110/70 mm Hg to a racing 180/110 mm Hg or higher. These changes occur without conscious thought and are directed by complex interactions among your central nervous system, hormones, and substances produced in your blood vessels.

Despite these natural fluctuations, your body keeps your blood pressure relatively stable most of the time. Just as a thermostat adjusts your furnace or air conditioner to keep your house at a comfortable temperature, pressure-sensing nerve cells in the cardiovascular system, called baroreceptors, continuously monitor your blood pressure. When blood pressure gets too high (such as during times of stress) or too low (when you're dehydrated, for example), baroreceptors relay this information to your autonomic nervous system, which sets off a chain of events designed to restore blood pressure to normal levels (see Figure 2, below). Sometimes the system falls short of the mark, however, leading to a problem known as orthostatic hypotension, particularly in the elderly (see "When blood pressure suddenly drops," page 6).

The inner wall of blood vessels, known as the endothelium, also plays a key role in regulating blood pressure. Far from being an inert conduit for blood flow, the endothelial lining secretes doz-

Figure 2: How key hormones affect blood pressure

Like an expert driver, the body constantly adjusts blood pressure in response to small changes in the environment. The central mechanism for regulating blood pressure involves a series of hormones and is known as the renin-angiotensin-aldosterone system. The interaction of these hormones takes place primarily in the circulatory system, the nervous system, and the kidneys. However, the renin-angiotensin system appears to operate independently within other organs, such as the brain and the blood vessels.

❶ When blood pressure falls, the nervous system sends a signal to the kidneys to release renin into the bloodstream. (The kidneys themselves also detect the reduction in blood pressure directly, stimulating additional release of renin, so the system works in two ways.) Renin splits angiotensinogen, a large protein in the bloodstream, to create angiotensin I.

❷ Angiotensin I is then converted into smaller pieces, including angiotensin II, which causes small arteries to constrict, thereby raising blood pressure.

❸ Angiotensin II also spurs the adrenal glands to release another hormone, aldosterone.

❹ Aldosterone causes the kidneys to retain sodium and water, which raises blood volume and blood pressure.

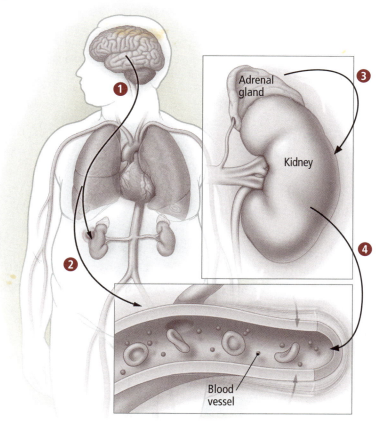

When blood pressure suddenly drops

If your blood pressure drops dramatically when you stand up, you have a condition known as orthostatic hypotension (hypotension means low blood pressure). This briefly reduces the amount of blood that reaches your brain, which can lead to dizziness, lightheadedness, and blurred vision. The higher your blood pressure is, the farther it can fall. However, people with orthostatic hypotension don't always have these symptoms, or they have them only occasionally. The problem may not be diagnosed until a person faints and falls.

About 30% of people ages 70 and older have orthostatic hypotension. One contributing factor is baroreceptors that become less sensitive with age and less able to respond rapidly. Older people are also more likely to take drugs that may worsen orthostatic hypotension. Common culprits include beta blockers (which reduce heart rate) and alpha blockers (used in men to treat an enlarged prostate). Cold and allergy drugs—especially diphenhydramine (Benadryl)—and most antidepressants can also contribute to the problem. In addition, people may lose their sense of thirst as they age, and dehydration makes the problem worse. Diabetes or other diseases, such as Parkinson's disease or cancer, may cause orthostatic hypotension as well.

Diagnosing the problem

Ask your doctor to measure your blood pressure after you've been sitting quietly or lying flat for five minutes, and again one and three minutes after you stand up. After you stand up, if your systolic pressure (the first number of the reading) falls more than 20 mm Hg or your diastolic pressure (the second number) drops at least 10 mm Hg, you may have orthostatic hypotension. You can also use a home blood pressure monitor to check your pressure first thing in the morning and throughout the day (especially after having a dizzy spell or taking medications).

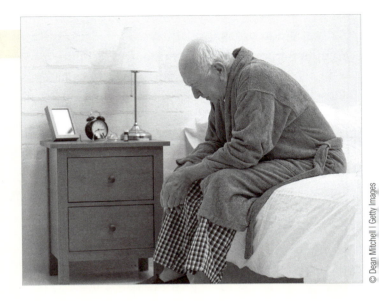

Dealing with dips

A range of strategies may help prevent episodes of low blood pressure. The first step should be a careful review of your medications with your doctor or a trusted pharmacist. The following suggestions may also help:

- **Focus on fluids.** Drink fluids throughout the day; don't wait until you're thirsty. But avoid alcohol, which can cause you to become dehydrated.

- **Support your legs or lower belly.** Compression stockings that squeeze the legs may help. Thigh-high or waist-high versions are best, because knee-high stockings may bunch and tighten, cutting off blood flow. A girdle-like abdominal binder that fastens with Velcro may also be helpful in extreme cases.

- **Get a leg up.** Getting out of bed is a common trigger, so pump your legs up and down a few times while you're still sitting on the edge of your bed to get your blood flowing. After you stand up, remain still for a moment to allow your body to adjust to the change in position.

ens of substances that interact with the circulating blood as well as with the cell layer that lies below it. Of particular significance for blood pressure are the vasodilators (nitric oxide and prostacyclin) and the vasoconstrictors (angiotensin II and endothelin-1). These chemical messengers instruct your blood vessels to widen or narrow based on your body's minute-by-minute blood flow requirements. As long as your blood pressure is in the normal range, healthy vessels tend to be dilated (wide). ♥

Types of high blood pressure

Physicians classify high blood pressure not only by how high it is (see Table 1, page 4) but also by its causes and characteristics. This determination may affect your treatment. Following are some of the most common types.

Essential hypertension

About 90% to 95% of people with high blood pressure have what's called essential hypertension. Also known as primary hypertension, this is high blood pressure that isn't caused by another medical condition, medication, or substance (see "Secondary hypertension," above right). Most experts believe a variety of factors contribute to the development of essential hypertension, many of them as yet unknown. If this is correct, it may explain why certain treatments lower blood pressure in some people, but not in others. For example, people who are salt-sensitive sometimes control their blood pressure with a low-sodium diet alone, while others find sodium intake has little or no influence on their blood pressure.

Isolated systolic hypertension

Essential hypertension may affect both systolic and diastolic pressure to a similar degree, or it can affect mainly systolic pressure. In the latter case, it's known as isolated systolic hypertension. This is the most common form of high blood pressure in the elderly.

In this case, the cause is clear. As people age, their arteries tend to lose elasticity and become less able to accommodate surges of blood. The damage created in the vessel lining when blood flows through the arteries at high pressure can accelerate the buildup of cholesterol-filled plaque inside arteries. Eventually, plaque deposits lead to atherosclerosis (hardening of the arteries), which in turn can elevate systolic blood pressure, while diastolic pressure stays in the normal range. Isolated systolic hypertension can be difficult to treat since there are no drugs that lower only systolic pressure.

Secondary hypertension

As its name implies, secondary hypertension arises from some other, often treatable, condition. These conditions are listed here, with the most common ones first.

Hyperaldosteronism

The leading cause of secondary hypertension is overproduction of aldosterone, the hormone made by the adrenal glands that helps the kidneys regulate potassium and sodium levels. This condition, called hyperaldosteronism, causes the body to retain sodium and lose potassium—which in turn leads to high blood pressure and fluid retention (see Figure 2, page 5). If a tumor in the adrenal gland is causing the overproduction, the treatment of choice is often surgery. In other cases, people with this condition need only to restrict their sodium intake and take a medication that blocks the action of aldosterone.

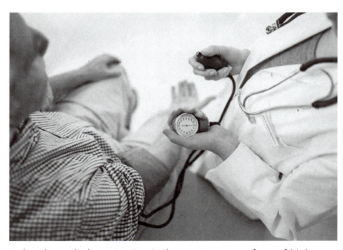

Isolated systolic hypertension is the most common form of high blood pressure in the elderly. In this condition, systolic blood pressure rises, while diastolic pressure remains normal.

Medications and other substances

Many medications, including some over-the-counter drugs, can elevate blood pressure. So can other substances, such as alcohol and caffeine as well as certain herbal supplements and recreational drugs. Table 2 (at right) lists the most common of these medications and substances and provides advice and (when applicable) alternative drugs or therapies. Among the most frequent offenders are the nonsteroidal anti-inflammatory drugs, or NSAIDs (see "Pain medications and heart risk," page 10).

The nasal decongestants found in most over-the-counter cold, flu, and allergy medicines and some weight-loss supplements can boost blood pressure and interfere with medications used to treat hypertension. Fortunately, some cold, cough, and flu remedies are specially formulated for people with high blood pressure, such as Coricidin HBP, which contains the decongestant chlorpheniramine. However, if you are taking a blood pressure drug, it's always a good idea to talk to your doctor before taking any over-the-counter medications.

Certain medications prescribed for autoimmune diseases—such as glucocorticoids (also called corticosteroids), cyclosporine, and tacrolimus—constrict blood vessels throughout the body, as do some drugs used to treat cancer. High blood pressure may also be a side effect of some drugs used to treat depression, including MAO inhibitors and tricyclic antidepressants.

Shortly after birth control pills came on the market in the 1960s, researchers discovered they could raise blood pressure, sometimes to dangerously high levels. As a result, they were found to increase a woman's risk of having a stroke, particularly among smokers. However, these early oral contraceptives contained considerably

Table 2: Frequently used medications and substances that can raise blood pressure

DRUG OR SUBSTANCE	ADVICE AND SUGGESTED ALTERNATIVES
Prescription medications	
Amphetamines amphetamine (Adzenys, Dyanvel, others) dexmethylphenidate (Focalin) dextroamphetamine (Dexadrine) methylphenidate (Concerta, Ritalin, others)	Discontinue or decrease dose. Consider behavioral therapies for ADHD.
Atypical antipsychotics clozapine (Clozaril, others) olanzapine (Zyprexa)	Discontinue or limit use when possible. Consider an alternative such as aripiprazole (Abilify) or ziprasidone (Geodon).
Cancer drugs bevacizumab (Avastin) sorafenif (Nexavar) sunitinib (Sutent)	Start or increase blood pressure medications.
Drugs for depression or other mood disorders monoamine oxidase inhibitors (MAOIs), such as isocarboxazid (Marplan) or phenelzine (Nardil) serotonin-norepinephrine reuptake inhibitors (SNRIs), such as duloxetine (Cymbalta) or venlafaxine (Effexor) tricyclic antidepressants (TCAs) such as amitriptyline (Elavil, others) or clomipramine (Anafranil)	Consider selective serotonin receptor inhibitors (SSRIs) as alternatives, such as sertraline (Zoloft) and citalopram (Celexa). Avoid tyramine-containing foods (such as aged cheese and cured meats) with MAOIs.
Immunosuppressants cyclosporine (Gengraf, others)	Consider switching to tacrolimus (Prograf), which may have fewer effects on blood pressure.
Oral contraceptives (birth control pills)	Use low-dose pills (no more than 20–30 mcg ethinyl estradiol); a progestin-only form of contraception; or barrier methods of birth control (such as condoms). Stop using an oral contraceptive if it causes high blood pressure. Avoid if you have uncontrolled hypertension.
Oral corticosteroids dexamethasone (Decadron) fludrocortisone (Florinef) methylprednisolone (Medrol) prednisolone (Flo-Pred, others) prednisone (Sterapred)	Avoid or limit use when possible. Consider inhaled or topical steroids when feasible.

continued on page 9

Table 2 continued from page 8	
DRUG OR SUBSTANCE	ADVICE AND SUGGESTED ALTERNATIVES
Over-the-counter medications	
Decongestants phenylephrine (Sudafed PE) pseudoephedrine (Sudafed)	Use for shortest duration possible; do not use if you have severe or uncontrolled hypertension. Consider nasal saline, intranasal corticosteroids, or antihistamines as appropriate.
Nonsteroidal anti-inflammatory drugs (NSAIDs) celecoxib (Celebrex); less likely than others in this category ibuprofen (Advil, Motrin) naproxen (Aleve, Naprosyn)	Consider alternative pain relievers, such as acetaminophen (Tylenol) or tramadol (Conzip, Ultram), or use topical NSAIDs such as diclofenac gel (Voltaren), depending on your specific needs.
Other substances	
Alcohol	Limit alcohol to one drink daily for women, two drinks daily for men.
Caffeine	Limit to less than 300 mg daily, or about the amount in three 8-ounce cups of coffee. Temporarily raises blood pressure in people with hypertension, but long-term use is not linked to high blood pressure or heart disease. Avoid if you have uncontrolled high blood pressure.
Herbal supplements ephedra (ma huang) St. John's wort in combination with MAOIs or yohimbine	Avoid using.
Licorice (found in candies, gum, and tea)	Limit to occasional use if you have high blood pressure.
Recreational drugs "bath salts" cocaine methamphetamine	Discontinue or avoid use.

Source: American College of Cardiology and American Heart Association, 2017 Guideline for the Prevention, Detection, Evaluation, and Management of High Blood Pressure in Adults.

higher doses of estrogen and progesterone than current formulations do. Today, it's much less common for oral contraceptives to increase blood pressure, and when it does happen, it's usually among women who smoke, are overweight or obese, or are over 35. In these cases, blood pressure usually returns to normal after the woman stops taking the pill.

In rare cases, certain toxic environmental substances, such as lead or cadmium, can cause hypertension.

Hyperthyroidism

The thyroid gland, a butterfly-shaped gland in the neck, produces hormones that control how the body uses energy. Many diseases and conditions, including Graves' disease or a benign tumor on the thyroid gland, can trigger an overproduction of thyroid hormone, known as hyperthyroidism. The condition can cause high blood pressure and a rapid heartbeat, as well as difficulty sleeping, heat intolerance, excess sweating, and weight loss. Treatment to suppress the gland's activity can resolve these symptoms, including restoring a normal blood pressure.

Renal artery stenosis

A common cause of secondary hypertension is renal artery stenosis, a narrowing of the arteries that supply the kidneys with blood (see Figure 3, page 11). This condition can occur as a result of a deposit of fatty material on the artery wall (atherosclerotic plaque) or, in young women, from an overgrowth of muscular tissue in the artery wall (fibromuscular dysplasia).

Some cases require bypass surgery, but most can be treated successfully by angioplasty. This procedure dilates the constricted artery with an inflatable balloon that's attached to a catheter. Angioplasty is simple, fast, and relatively painless.

Angioplasty begins with a small incision in an artery near the groin. From there, the physician threads the catheter through the blood vessels to the narrowed artery, using fluoroscopic (x-ray–like) images projected on a monitor as a guide. After opening the artery with the balloon, the physician usually inserts a stent, a wire mesh tube that widens the channel. Even after the blockage is cleared, however, blood pressure might not return to normal.

> ### Pain medications and heart risk
>
> The common pain relievers known as nonsteroidal anti-inflammatory drugs (NSAIDs) are widely used to ease pain, quell inflammation, and cool fevers. They include aspirin, ibuprofen (Advil, Motrin), naproxen (Aleve, Naprosyn), and the prescription drug celecoxib (Celebrex). Today, all NSAIDs except aspirin are suspected of raising heart attack risk, prompting the FDA to mandate a warning about this side effect on all NSAID labels. Celecoxib appears to be less dangerous than the other NSAIDs.
>
> NSAIDs tend to raise blood pressure, probably by altering blood flow in the kidneys, causing the body to retain more sodium and water. They may also change levels of substances in the blood that make clots more likely. A blood clot can block a narrowed artery in the heart, triggering a heart attack.
>
> If you have high blood pressure, be cautious about using NSAIDs. If you need to take painkillers for an injury or a chronic condition like arthritis, consider other alternatives first, such as heating pads, ice, or physical therapy, if appropriate. Next, try aspirin or acetaminophen (Tylenol). Keep in mind that acetaminophen can damage the liver, especially in people who drink alcohol. With any pain reliever, always take the lowest possible dose for the shortest possible time.

Pheochromocytoma

A rare, usually noncancerous tumor called a pheochromocytoma secretes excessive amounts of epinephrine and norepinephrine, which constrict most arteries and raise blood pressure. Other symptoms may include tremors, palpitations, sweating, nervousness, headache, weight loss, and fainting. Treatment consists of medications that block the hormones' effects and surgery to remove the tumor. Pheochromocytomas are typically confined to the adrenal glands, which lie on top of the kidneys. However, about 10% spread beyond the adrenals or arise at other sites in the body. If a surgeon cannot remove the tumor, radiation or chemotherapy may be necessary.

Cushing's syndrome

Cushing's syndrome is a hormonal disorder characterized by a high level of circulating cortisol, a hormone produced by the adrenal glands. The disorder can cause high blood pressure, as well as weight gain, swelling of the face, excessive body hair, acne, osteoporosis, diabetes, and a fatty deposit on the upper back called a buffalo hump. Cushing's syndrome may be caused by excessive synthesis of cortisol by the adrenal gland, or by a person's taking corticosteroid drugs for extended periods to treat severe allergy or autoimmune disorders. In the first case, treatment generally involves drug therapy or surgery. In the second, attempts are made to reduce the corticosteroid dosage.

Coarctation of the aorta

The aorta is the body's largest artery. Coarctation is a rare birth defect in which a segment of the aorta, usually in the chest, is abnormally narrow. This condition, which may not be discovered until adulthood, moderately increases blood pressure in the arms, while blood pressure in the legs is considerably lower. Often, pulses in the groin and legs are very weak or altogether absent. Symptoms include headache, fatigue, leg weakness, and poor circulation in the legs. Inserting a wire mesh tube (stent) that keeps the narrowed segment of the artery open usually alleviates the symptoms of limited blood flow, but high blood pressure often persists.

Sleep apnea

About a third of people with high blood pressure suffer from sleep apnea, a condition in which changes in the throat during sleep cause repeated interruptions to breathing. It is often associated with obesity and resolves if the person loses weight. Sleep apnea sufferers actually stop breathing from 15 to more than 100 times an hour. Each pause causes oxygen levels to drop. The body responds by releasing epinephrine (also called adrenaline), a stress hormone. When this happens over and over, adrenaline levels remain high. This can lead to high blood pressure.

White-coat hypertension

Stress can elevate blood pressure. For this reason, some people whose blood pressure is usually normal can have high blood pressure in the doctor's office. This phenomenon is dubbed white-coat hypertension. In the past, doctors often dismissed these elevated readings as a reflection of the temporary anxiety many people experience at the clinic or hospital. But now some experts think white-coat hypertension is worth investigating because it might shed light on how stress influences blood pressure.

People who are habitually affected by stress—whether from losing a job, feeling pressure at work, or simply getting stuck in traffic—may develop temporary or longer-lasting high blood pressure that could inflict some of the same damage as having it full-time. By figuring out how these people's blood pressure varies throughout the day, doctors can determine how best to treat them—if at all.

To get this information, a person periodically checks his or her blood pressure at home over the course of a week or two (see "Monitoring blood pressure at home," page 22).

Masked hypertension

Masked hypertension is the opposite of white-coat hypertension: your blood pressure reading is normal at the doctor's office but high at other times—sometimes as a result of daily stressors, sometimes as a result of lifestyle factors such as smoking. It's hard to know just how common it is, since doctors don't routinely tell people to measure their blood pressure at home if it's normal in the doctor's office. The only reason we know it exists is from clinical studies that required people to undergo ambulatory blood pressure monitoring (see "Around-the-clock monitoring," page 22). In these studies, anywhere from 10% to 40% of the participants were found to have masked hypertension, depending on the exact population evaluated. Compared with people who have normal blood pressure, those with masked hypertension may face a higher risk of stroke and other cardiovascular problems (although not as high a risk as in those with sustained high blood pressure).

Labile hypertension

Labile means ever-changing, and in labile hypertension, blood pressure fluctuates far more than usual. Your blood pressure might soar from 119/76 mm Hg at 10 a.m. to 170/104 mm Hg at 4 p.m. These fluctuations can spring from a variety of sources, such as too much caffeine, anxiety attacks, or stress. Whatever the cause, these transient episodes of high blood pressure can be dangerous and should be treated. Home blood pressure monitoring over a 24-hour period helps determine the best treatment strategy (see "Around-the-clock monitoring," page 22). You're most likely to experience labile hypertension before sustained high blood pressure becomes apparent, thus making it hard to diagnose. Its duration can range from a few weeks to many years.

Resistant hypertension

Hypertension is often treated by adopting healthier habits and taking drugs to lower blood pressure. The first drug prescribed, however, doesn't always work. Your doctor may have to increase the dose, prescribe an additional drug, or substitute a different drug. Sometimes, in spite of these efforts, blood pressure

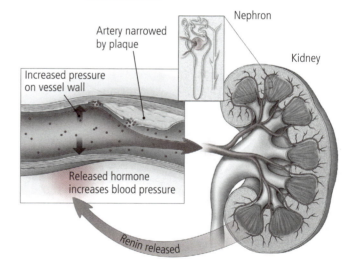

Figure 3: The kidney–blood pressure connection

Blood flows to the kidneys through the renal arteries, which branch into successively smaller blood vessels, finally ending in small clusters of capillaries known as glomeruli. Each cluster, or glomerulus, is part of a nephron—a tube-like structure that filters and purifies the blood. If the arteries that feed blood to the kidneys are narrowed—a condition known as renal artery stenosis—the body reacts by producing renin, a hormone that causes small arteries to narrow further. This kicks off a cycle of even higher blood pressure and resultant kidney damage. Over time, the diminished blood flow can damage or destroy the nephrons. When this happens, the kidney cannot filter wastes properly.

remains persistently high. Resistant hypertension is defined as blood pressure that remains stubbornly high even when a person is taking three or more blood pressure drugs (at least one of which is a diuretic) at the highest doses he or she can tolerate. It occurs in about one in 10 people with hypertension.

In some instances, resistant hypertension results from drug interactions. For example, blood pressure drugs may lose their effectiveness if you're also taking certain antidepressants or even some over-the-counter drugs, such as pain relievers and decongestants (see Table 2, page 8). Drinking too much alcohol can also contribute to high blood pressure. Another culprit is licorice, found in candy as well as some chewing gums, breath fresheners, and herbal teas. Other causes include panic attacks, chronic pain, sleep apnea, fluid retention, kidney damage, weight gain, and inflammatory artery disease (arteritis). But the most common reasons are consuming too much sodium or not complying with the treatment regimen.

Give your doctor as much information as possible about the medications you take (including herbal remedies and nutritional supplements), the foods and drinks you consume, and any conditions you may have. There are often simple ways to avoid the interactions that make blood pressure medications ineffective.

Malignant hypertension

Although rare, malignant hypertension is the most ominous form of high blood pressure. It's marked by an unusually sudden rise in blood pressure to dangerous levels, often with the diastolic reading reaching 130 mm Hg or higher. However, it may also occur at lower, seemingly more normal blood pressure levels if the rise is particularly abrupt. Unlike other kinds of hypertension, it's accompanied by dramatic symptoms such as severe headache, shortness of breath, chest pain, nausea and vomiting, blurred vision or even blindness, seizures, and loss of consciousness.

Malignant hypertension is a medical emergency. It places people at immediate risk for heart attack, stroke, and heart failure or death. It can also cause acute liver failure. Anyone who develops the condition must be hospitalized immediately.

Malignant hypertension develops in less than 1% of people who already have high blood pressure. In rare cases, the appearance of malignant hypertension is the first sign that a person has high blood pressure. While the cause of this condition is unknown, you should never stop taking blood pressure medication without your doctor's supervision. Doing so might cause a precipitous increase in your blood pressure.

Hypertension during pregnancy

Between 5% and 8% of all pregnant women in the United States develop high blood pressure. Pregnancy-induced hypertension may appear as early as the 20th week of pregnancy and occasionally as late as one week after delivery. When elevated blood pressure is accompanied by an excess of protein in the urine, the condition is known as pre-eclampsia. In most women who develop hypertension during pregnancy, blood pressure returns to normal within six months after they give birth.

The causes of pregnancy-induced hypertension and pre-eclampsia are unknown. Signs of pre-eclampsia, in addition to protein in the urine, include swelling of the hands and face and blood-clotting abnormalities. For most women, pre-eclampsia never proceeds beyond the mild stage. For some women, though, the disease develops rapidly, moving from mild to severe in a matter of weeks or sometimes days. Doctors usually recommend bed rest. But if the problem remains or worsens, hospitalization and medications are often necessary to prevent pre-eclampsia from progressing to eclampsia, a serious medical condition. The medications that can be used are limited because of concerns about harm to the fetus. Eclampsia, which is characterized by dangerously high blood pressure and seizures, can cause coma and even the death of the mother, the baby, or both. Since eclampsia frequently disappears once the baby is born, doctors often induce labor. They may also prescribe anticonvulsant medications. If a woman still has high blood pressure after giving birth, she may need medication. Little is known about the effects of blood pressure drugs in breast milk, however, so breastfed infants must be closely monitored.

What puts you at risk for high blood pressure?

Essential hypertension has no clear cause. As a result, identifying risk factors can be difficult. Researchers have discovered certain patterns, however. Some factors are things you have no control over—for example, you can't alter your genes. But others, like smoking and heavy drinking, are habits you can change.

Risk factors you can't control

Even though you can't control these risks, that doesn't mean you can forget about them. Awareness of your risk factors can help you put your overall cardiovascular risk profile into perspective and may provide you with extra incentive to adopt healthier habits.

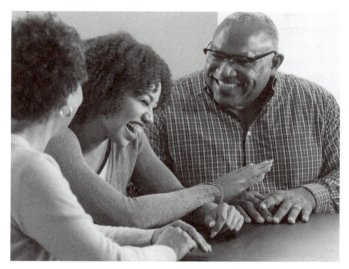

Hypertension tends to run in families, in part because of genetic vulnerabilities. African Americans often develop it earlier and to a greater degree than do people of other races.

Family history

Like many disorders, high blood pressure tends to run in families. In addition, a family history of heart attack, stroke, diabetes, kidney disease, or high cholesterol increases a person's risk of developing high blood pressure.

This doesn't necessarily mean that genetics always plays a role. Some of the similarities observed in families may be the result of environmental influences. Children's eating patterns, coping skills, and propensity toward healthy and unhealthy habits are shaped by their parents' behavior and the social climate in which they're raised.

A significant percentage of essential hypertension cases that occur in families and up to 65% of cases in pairs of twins may have a genetic basis. To date, researchers have identified dozens of gene sites associated with high blood pressure. Some are rare variants of genes that provide instructions for making proteins involved in relaxing blood vessels and eliminating excess sodium from the body. Other variants are linked to both high blood pressure and damage to tissue in the heart and blood vessels.

Age

Although aging doesn't invariably lead to high blood pressure, hypertension becomes more common in later years. Diastolic pressure increases gradually over the years by about 10 mm Hg until age 55 in men and 60 in women, at which time it begins to decline. Between ages 30 and 65, systolic pressure increases an average of 20 mm Hg, and it continues to climb after 70. This age-associated increase largely explains isolated systolic hypertension (see page 7).

Gender

Up to about age 55, women are less likely than men to develop high blood pressure. But women's blood pressures, especially the systolic readings, rise more sharply after that. Indeed, after age 55, women are at greater risk for high blood pressure. This pattern may be partly explained by hormonal differences between the sexes. Estrogen tends to protect women against hypertension, but as the production of estrogen drops with menopause, women lose its beneficial effects, and their blood pressures climb.

What is salt sensitivity?

Sodium does not affect everyone the same way. Some people are described as salt-sensitive, meaning they have an increase of 10 mm Hg or more in blood pressure when going from a low-sodium to a high-sodium diet. But being salt-sensitive does not necessarily mean you have high blood pressure. About one-quarter to one-third of Americans with *normal* blood pressure meet that definition—although they may go on to develop high blood pressure later, since salt sensitivity increases with age and weight gain. Among people with high blood pressure, fully half are salt-sensitive.

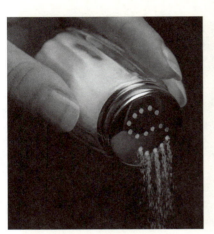

Half of people with high blood pressure are salt-sensitive, meaning that their blood pressure rises by 10 mm Hg with a high-sodium diet.

Genetics also appears to play a role. Among African Americans, the proportion who are salt-sensitive rises to 75%. Some researchers suspect that over the course of many generations, people who lived in equatorial Africa developed a genetic predisposition to retain sodium in their bodies. This can be beneficial in a hot, dry climate because it allows the body to conserve water. However, in a more temperate climate, sodium retention causes the body to hold on to more water than it needs. That increases blood volume, which, in turn, raises blood pressure. Generations later, the American descendants of these individuals remain disproportionately salt-sensitive.

Unfortunately, formal testing for salt sensitivity is laborious and costly. It involves first increasing the sodium in your diet, then severely restricting it, while continuously measuring how much sodium leaves your body in urine—all during a three-day hospital stay.

But an official diagnosis of salt sensitivity would not change your treatment. Doctors still use the same medications and advise the same sodium limits for all people with high blood pressure, regardless of their sensitivity to salt—in part because too much dietary salt negates the benefits of many blood pressure drugs.

Race

African Americans often develop high blood pressure earlier and to a greater degree than do people of other races. Genetics may be at least partially to blame (see "What is salt sensitivity?" at left). Although African American adults are 40% more likely to have high blood pressure than their white counterparts, they are significantly less likely to have the condition under control.

Controllable risk factors

Your health habits are key factors in determining your cardiovascular risk. In fact, you may be able to overcome the effects of other risk factors and bring your blood pressure readings into a safe range simply by making changes in your lifestyle, such as quitting smoking, reducing your salt intake, and losing weight (for more detailed explanations, see "Lifestyle changes to lower your blood pressure," page 23).

Obesity

Excess weight and hypertension often go hand in hand, because carrying even a few extra pounds forces your heart to work harder. Being overweight increases the risk of high blood pressure approximately threefold. The risk continues to rise as body mass index progresses into the obesity range. By contrast, systolic and diastolic blood pressures drop an average of 1 mm Hg for roughly every pound or two of weight lost, although the actual amount varies widely from person to person.

Sedentary lifestyle

Compared with people who are physically active, those who are sedentary are significantly more likely to develop hypertension and suffer heart attacks. Like any muscle, your heart gets stronger with exercise. A stronger heart pumps more blood more efficiently, with less force, through your body. Other cardiovascular benefits of exercise include increasing levels of "good" HDL cholesterol and making stroke-causing clots less likely.

Smoking

Doctors have long known that smoking promotes heart disease, but for a long time smoking didn't appear to have a direct connection to hypertension. That is no longer the case. Doctors now know that the nicotine in tobacco stimulates the central nervous system. Whether you smoke a cigarette, chew tobacco, or absorb nicotine from a patch, your body responds by releasing a stress hormone called epinephrine (adrenaline), which increases your heart rate and blood pressure, both while you're smoking and for some time afterward.

Excess salt

Doctors first noticed a link between hypertension and table salt—that is, sodium chloride, the most common form of dietary sodium—in the early 1900s, when they found that restricting salt in people with kidney failure and severe hypertension brought their blood pressures down and improved their kidney function. When a massive effort began in the 1960s to educate the public about lowering the risk of heart disease, one recommendation was that all Americans reduce salt consumption to prevent hypertension. However, rather than decreasing, the average amount of sodium in the American diet has risen, likely as the result of our growing reliance on salt-laden processed and prepared foods.

Heavy drinking

Having three or more drinks in one sitting temporarily increases your blood pressure. Over time, excessive drinking—including binge drinking—can have longer-lasting detrimental effects on blood pressure. (Binge drinking is defined as drinking enough to attain a blood alcohol level of 0.08%, which typically happens when a man has five or more drinks or a woman has four or more within about a two-hour span.) Heavy drinking can interfere with blood pressure medications and may also boost the risk of stroke and heart failure.

How high blood pressure harms your health

Although high blood pressure seldom produces symptoms, the intense pounding of blood associated with it gradually and stealthily damages artery walls. Small arteries are especially vulnerable. The walls respond by thickening and losing their elasticity and strength. As a result, less blood can pass through them, depriving surrounding tissues of oxygen and nutrients. The vessel walls are also more prone to rupture. Eventually, high blood pressure damages not just the blood vessels themselves, but also the heart, brain, kidneys, and eyes. These are the "target organs" of high blood pressure (see Figure 4, page 17). The longer you have high blood pressure, the greater your chances of developing serious disorders such as heart disease, stroke, kidney disease, and loss of vision.

African Americans are particularly at risk: not only are they more likely to develop high blood pressure, but they are also more apt to suffer from its complications. African Americans with hypertension have higher rates of stroke, heart disease, kidney disease, and diabetes than whites who have hypertension. African Americans are also more likely than whites to die as a result of high blood pressure.

Stroke

Untreated high blood pressure is the leading cause of stroke, which is the fourth leading killer in the United States. Two-thirds of people having a first stroke have blood pressures that are higher than 160/95 mm Hg.

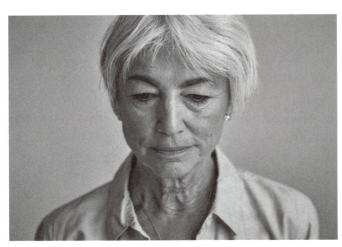

The longer you have high blood pressure, the greater your chances of developing serious disorders such as heart disease, stroke, kidney disease, dementia, and loss of vision.

If your blood pressure is 160/95 mm Hg, you're about four times more likely to have a stroke than someone with normal blood pressure.

High blood pressure can lead to either of the two types of stroke: ischemic stroke, which is caused by a blockage of an artery that nourishes the brain, and hemorrhagic stroke, which occurs when a vessel in or near the brain ruptures.

More than 80% of strokes are ischemic, and atherosclerosis plays an important role in most of these cases. Atherosclerosis is the thickening of the inner layer of artery walls from the buildup of plaque—deposits of fat, cholesterol, and dead cells. This buildup narrows the passageway, diminishing or obstructing blood flow (see Figure 5, page 18). An ischemic stroke occurs when blood supply to part of the brain is cut off by either a clot that has developed inside a brain artery (thrombosis) or a clot that has been swept into the brain artery from somewhere else in the body (embolism).

High blood pressure is one cause of the initial damage that leads to atherosclerosis. Increased blood pressure damages the vessel walls, causing inflammation. This inflammation, in turn, encourages plaque buildup and narrowing of the arteries. High blood pressure may also increase substances that make blood "sticky" and more apt to form stroke-causing clots.

In a hemorrhagic stroke, the walls of small arteries become weakened and eventually burst, causing blood to leak into a portion of the brain, ultimately damaging or destroying it. Because high blood pressure is the most frequent cause of weakened vessel walls, hemorrhagic stroke is most likely to occur in people with high blood pressure. Although every stroke is dangerous, hemorrhagic events are often the most devastating.

A stroke's severity depends on which part of the brain is affected and how large the damaged area is. A mild stroke may cause few or no lasting problems. But approximately one-third of major strokes are fatal, and another third cause permanent damage, such as weakness or paralysis on one side of the body, vision disturbances, impaired speech, and diminished intellect.

Cardiovascular disease

By making your blood vessel walls more susceptible to atherosclerosis, high blood pressure increases not only your likelihood of having a stroke, but also your risk of having a heart attack. When coronary arteries become completely blocked—either by a clot resulting from a ruptured plaque or by debris such as fats, cholesterol, and dead cells—a heart attack results.

Fragments from these deposits, called emboli, can also break away from large blood vessels such as the aorta, travel through the bloodstream, and eventually block other vessels, such as those supplying the legs (causing circulatory problems) or the brain (causing a stroke). Having high cholesterol in addition to high blood pressure exacerbates this process and increases your risk of cardiovascular complications.

In addition to making atherosclerosis more likely, high blood pressure also forces the heart to work increasingly harder to drive blood through the body. As a result, the left ventricle, the heart's main pumping chamber, becomes thicker and more muscular in order to contract with greater force. This compensation—known as left ventricular hypertrophy—eventually becomes counterproductive. As the heart muscle enlarges, it needs progressively more oxygen, but the coronary arteries, which are also thickened and narrowed as a result of hypertension, become less able to deliver it. The lack of oxygen can cause angina (chest pain) and, if severe enough, a heart attack.

The combination of left ventricular hypertrophy and diseased coronary arteries—spurred on by high blood pressure—may also lead to heart failure (the inability of your heart to pump blood efficiently throughout your body). In fact, if you have uncontrolled high blood pressure, you're twice as likely to develop heart failure as someone with normal blood pressure. Unlike your biceps muscles, which grow both larger and stronger when you lift weights, increased thickness of your heart muscle doesn't translate into strength. As your blood supply fails to keep up with the muscle's growth, your heart weakens, and this in turn can lead to either of the two primary kinds of heart failure. Heart failure with reduced ejection fraction arises when your heart cannot pump forcefully enough to push a sufficient amount of blood into circulation. Heart failure with preserved ejection fraction occurs when your heart can't properly fill with blood because it's stiff and has trouble relaxing. Symptoms of heart failure include weakness and fatigue (because your muscles aren't getting enough

Figure 4: Danger zones

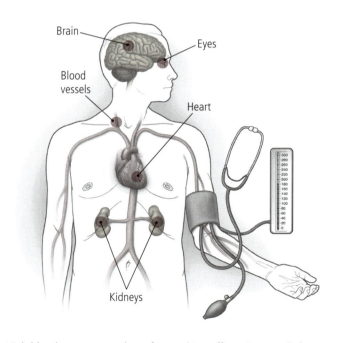

High blood pressure can have far-reaching effects. It not only harms the arteries and blood vessels, making them stiffer and narrower, but can also damage the heart, brain, eyes, and kidneys—which, for this reason, are known as the "target organs" of hypertension.

blood), shortness of breath, and fluid buildup (known as edema) in your lungs, feet, ankles, and legs.

Atrial fibrillation

Longstanding, uncontrolled high blood pressure is the most common cause of the heart rhythm disorder known as atrial fibrillation. People with atrial fibrillation experience periodic spells during which the upper chambers of their hearts quiver erratically. As a result, blood swirls around and pools inside the upper chambers, which may form clots that can cause a stroke if they break loose and make their way to the brain. Experts estimate that atrial fibrillation, which is most common among people over age 65, increases the risk of stroke about fivefold. In the Framingham Heart Study, atrial fibrillation was blamed for one of every four strokes among people over 80. Taking medications that prevent blood clotting (anticoagulants), such as warfarin, rivaroxaban (Xarelto), dabigatran (Pradaxa), or apixaban (Eliquis), can reduce the risk of stroke by more than two-thirds in people who have atrial fibrillation as well as other stroke risk factors. However, treatment with any anticoagulant carries risks of its own, including the risk of severe bleeding.

Figure 5: How plaque buildup narrows arteries

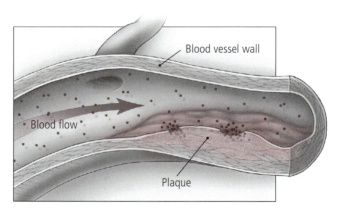

High blood pressure can lead to inflammation of the walls of your arteries, which in turn encourages fatty and fibrous substances to accumulate. As this debris—known as plaque—is deposited inside artery walls, your arteries become narrower and blood flow is reduced. This thickening of artery walls is called atherosclerosis.

Dementia

By accelerating atherosclerosis, high blood pressure can contribute to dementia—a loss of memory and thinking skills that interferes with daily life. Atherosclerosis impairs circulation, and a lack of blood supply can produce areas of dead tissue in the brain. Each incident of damage—which is actually a tiny stroke—affects such a small area of the brain that you may not notice any symptoms until a substantial amount of tissue has been destroyed. This condition, known as vascular dementia, is a well-recognized cause of memory loss in older people.

The link between vascular dementia and hypertension escaped notice for many years because people suffering from dementia often have normal or low blood pressure. But long-term studies now show that high blood pressure in midlife may predict poorer brain function in old age. Even slightly elevated blood pressure in middle age has been linked to a 30% higher risk of dementia two decades later.

High blood pressure also appears to harm memory by damaging the brain's white matter, the bundles of nerve fibers that connect brain cells. Changes in white matter occur to some degree in virtually everyone over age 60 and contribute to normal age-related memory loss. But damage to white matter is more extensive among people with high blood pressure. The good news: controlling blood pressure can lower the risk of dementia and slow its progression in people who already have it.

Kidney disease

Your kidneys are two bean-shaped organs, each about the size of a fist, that filter waste from the bloodstream. They also play a crucial role in the body's natural control of blood pressure by regulating the amount of water and sodium in circulation. When blood pressure rises, the kidneys excrete water and sodium. This action helps bring pressure back down by stimulating the loss of body fluids (through urination, for example), thereby reducing the volume of circulating blood. By contrast, when blood pressure falls, the kidneys retain water and sodium to conserve blood volume and raise pressure. People with high blood

High blood pressure and diabetes: A dangerous combination

More than three out of four adults with diabetes have blood pressure above 130/80 or are taking blood pressure drugs. Like high blood pressure, diabetes increases your chances of having a heart attack or stroke. Having both diabetes and hypertension raises these risks even more.

Although blood pressure and diabetes seem to be linked, the mechanism by which they interact is unclear. Some experts believe the common denominator may be problems stemming from the body's production and use of insulin. People with both type 2 diabetes and coronary artery disease frequently have too much circulating insulin (a problem called hyperinsulinemia). Excess insulin is thought to raise blood pressure in two ways: by causing the kidneys to retain sodium, and by prompting the sympathetic nervous system to release chemicals that constrict blood vessels.

Over time, most people with diabetes develop cardiovascular problems. Between 65% and 75% of people with diabetes will die from some type of cardiovascular disease—a death rate that is two to four times that of people without diabetes. Keeping blood pressure in check may be a vital factor in preventing heart disease and strokes among people with diabetes.

Not only are diabetes and high blood pressure linked to cardiovascular disease, but they can also lead to kidney disease and eye damage. That makes careful control of these conditions even more crucial.

Because of the increased risks associated with high blood pressure in people with diabetes, the new blood pressure guidelines advise medication for people with diabetes or chronic kidney disease if their blood pressure is 130/80 or greater. Two diabetes medications—empagliflozin (Jardiance) and liraglutide (Victoza)—have also been shown to lower the risk of serious complications and death from cardiovascular disease.

---

pressure tend to retain too much water and sodium.

Sustained high blood pressure damages the glomeruli, structures in the kidneys that filter waste products, sodium, and water from the bloodstream (see Figure 3, page 11). This damage is one of the most common causes of kidney failure. People with kidney failure (known medically as renal failure) become bloated with excessive fluid and weakened by the accumulation of toxic chemicals that are normally removed by the kidneys and excreted in urine. Uncontrolled high blood pressure is second only to diabetes as a cause of kidney failure, accounting for about one in four new cases.

Eye damage

The eye works by focusing visual images onto the retina, a sheet of nerve tissue at the back of the eyeball. Immediately behind the retina lies a network of tiny blood vessels that keeps this tissue richly supplied with oxygen and nutrients. High blood pressure can cause these arteries to narrow or break and bleed into the retina. It can also lead to swelling of the optic nerve, which carries images to the brain. Most people with this problem do not have symptoms, although they may experience headaches and vision problems. Longstanding, untreated high blood pressure can lead to loss of vision and even blindness.

Diagnosing high blood pressure

Because high blood pressure has no warning signs, you might easily be unaware you have it, at least until trouble strikes. That's why it's important to have your doctor check your blood pressure periodically. If you have high blood pressure, you should have it measured whenever you see any health care professional.

Measuring blood pressure

To determine whether you have hypertension, a medical professional will take a blood pressure reading. How you prepare for the test, the position of your arm, and other factors can change a blood pressure reading by 10% or more. That could be enough to hide high blood pressure, start you on a drug you don't really need, or lead your doctor to incorrectly adjust your medications.

National and international guidelines offer specific instructions for measuring blood pressure. If a doctor, nurse, or medical assistant isn't doing it right, don't hesitate to ask him or her to get with the guidelines.

Here's what you can do to ensure a correct reading:
- Don't drink a caffeinated beverage or smoke during the 30 minutes before the test.
- Sit quietly for five minutes before the test begins.
- During the measurement, sit in a chair with your feet on the floor and your arm supported so your elbow is at about heart level.
- The inflatable part of the cuff should completely cover at least 80% of your upper arm, and the cuff should be placed on bare skin, not over a shirt.
- Don't talk during the measurement.
- Have your blood pressure measured twice, with a brief break in between. If the readings are different by 5 points or more, have it done a third time.

There are times to break these rules. If you sometimes feel lightheaded when getting out of bed in the morning or when you stand after sitting, you should have your blood pressure checked while seated and then while standing to see if it falls when you change position (see "When blood pressure suddenly drops," page 6).

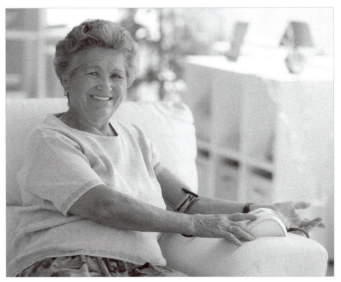

Taking your blood pressure regularly at home can give you a truer picture than a single reading in the doctor's office.

Because blood pressure varies throughout the day, your doctor will rarely diagnose hypertension on the basis of a single reading. Instead, he or she will want to confirm the measurements on at least two occasions, usually within a few weeks of one another. The exception to this rule is if you have a blood pressure reading of 160/100 mm Hg or higher, especially if there are symptoms of an underlying disease. A result this high calls for prompt treatment.

It's also a good idea to have your blood pressure measured in both arms at least once, since the reading in one arm may be higher (usually the right, since there's more direct blood flow from the heart on that side). The higher number should be used to make treatment decisions.

In general, blood pressures between 160/100 mm Hg and 179/109 mm Hg should be rechecked within one to two weeks, while measurements between 140/90 and 159/99 should be repeated within four weeks. Those with Stage 1 hypertension (systolic pressure of 130 to 139 or diastolic of 80 to 89) should be rechecked within four to six weeks. People in the elevated category (systolic pressure of 120 to 129 and diastolic less than 80 mm Hg) should be rechecked within four to six months, and those with a normal reading (less than 120/80 mm Hg) should be rechecked annually. However, your doctor may schedule a follow-up visit sooner if your previous blood pressure measurements were considerably lower; if signs of damage to the heart, brain, kidneys, or eyes are present; or if you have other cardiovascular risk factors. Also, most doctors routinely check your blood pressure whenever you go in for an office visit.

Gathering more data

After a high initial reading, it's often beneficial to have one or more measurements done outside the doctor's office before returning for the follow-up visit. This information can help your doctor distinguish between sustained and white-coat hypertension. Home monitoring can aid in the diagnosis, and doctors often suggest that people with high blood pressure learn to monitor their pressure at home (see "Monitoring blood pressure at home," page 22).

Once a diagnosis of hypertension is confirmed, the next steps are to determine whether damage to the heart, brain, kidneys, or eyes has occurred and to rule out any disorder that could be to blame for your high blood pressure (see "Secondary hypertension," page 7). Expect to undergo a thorough evaluation, including a medical history, physical examination, laboratory tests, and possibly other diagnostic exams such as a chest x-ray, echocardiogram, or exercise stress test. Mention any recent changes that could increase your risks for high blood pressure—including weight gain, increases in alcohol consumption or tobacco use, or reductions in physical activity. Also, list all your current and recent use of prescription and over-the-counter medications, dietary supplements, and even illegal drugs. Some of the substances found in these products can raise blood pressure or interfere with blood pressure medication.

Helpful medical tests

Routine urine and blood analyses can reveal medical conditions. For instance, protein or blood in the urine may be a sign of kidney damage, while glucose in the urine suggests diabetes. Blood tests typically measure sodium, potassium, chloride, calcium, bicarbonate, glucose, and cholesterol, as well as urea nitrogen or creatinine, which are indicators of kidney function. If your doctor suspects that you have another condition or evidence of damage to the heart, brain, kidneys, or eyes, he or she may recommend additional tests.

An electrocardiogram (ECG), which measures electrical activity of the heart and gives a general picture of the heart's health, is especially important. The initial ECG is called a baseline. Later ECGs can be compared with the original to reveal changes in heart rhythm or signs of coronary artery disease or thickening of the heart wall.

An exercise stress test assesses how your cardiovascular system responds to physical activity. If you have high blood pressure, this information is sometimes important to know before you start an exercise program. The test monitors the electrical activity of your heart and your blood pressure during exercise, which usually involves pedaling a stationary bike or walking on a treadmill. Stress tests can reveal problems that aren't apparent when you're at rest. In many circumstances, imaging scans of the heart's blood supply are done during stress testing.

Chest pain, dizzy spells, palpitations, or other symptoms may indicate some form of heart disease, which calls for additional testing. For instance, you may need Holter monitoring, in which you wear a portable device that takes a continuous ECG recording for 24 hours or longer. Another test is the echocardiogram, which uses ultrasound waves to show your heart in motion. It's used to diagnose thickening of the heart wall, valve defects, blood clots, and excessive fluid around the heart.

Symptoms such as urinary tract infections, frequent urination, or pain in your flank (low down on the side of your abdomen) may be signs of a kidney disorder. If the doctor hears a bruit—the sound of a rush of blood—through a stethoscope placed on the flank, it may be a sign of renal artery stenosis, a narrowing of an artery supplying the kidney (see Figure 3, page 11). You may have to undergo blood analyses and imaging tests to learn whether a kidney problem is causing your hypertension.

Monitoring blood pressure at home

Stress, exercise, and even a few drinks the night before your doctor's appointment can push your blood pressure up. So it's often difficult to tell whether an unusually high reading at the doctor's office means you have high blood pressure—or, if you have already been diagnosed with hypertension, that it's worsening—or whether a work deadline has temporarily inflated your numbers.

To offset this problem, many doctors encourage people to monitor blood pressure on their own. Home monitoring is especially useful for people with white-coat, masked, or labile hypertension, as well as to track responses to exercise, medications, or changes in treatment. It gives a more accurate idea of your blood pressure. It can help fine-tune the strategy for keeping your blood pressure in check. And it just might make you more invested in controlling a problem that has no symptoms until it spawns a heart attack or stroke or leads to heart or kidney failure.

At some point, be sure to check your machine against the one in your doctor's office. To get the most accurate blood pressure reading, follow the recommendations under "Measuring blood pressure" on page 20.

When you first start to check your blood pressure at home, measure it early in the morning, before you have taken your blood pressure pills, and again in the evening, every day for a week. After that, follow the plan your doctor recommends. And don't panic if one reading is high. Keep in mind that your blood pressure changes constantly throughout the day.

Many blood pressure meters store a week's worth of readings, or more. If yours doesn't, keep a record so you can show your doctor. There are some apps that will do this for you. Some even take the readings directly from the monitor, so that you don't need to write them down.

Doctors warn, however, that home blood pressure monitoring can become too much of a good thing. Just as getting on the scale several times a day is counterproductive when it comes to losing weight, overly frequent monitoring can create anxiety over small fluctuations without contributing to long-term blood pressure management.

Choosing and using a home blood pressure monitor

Most pharmacies have machines that customers can use free of charge, but a home monitor is more practical for taking daily readings. Your doctor may be able to lend you a blood pressure monitoring unit temporarily. If you need to buy the equipment for long-term use, your insurance plan may cover the expense.

There are dozens of home blood pressure monitors on the market, ranging in price from about $40 to $100. For best accuracy and ease of use, buy one with a cuff for the upper arm that automatically inflates and that automatically records the pressure. Models that store readings for a week or two can simplify record keeping. Be sure to choose one with the correct cuff size—the inflatable part should completely cover at least 80% of your bare upper arm. (If the cuff is too small, you can get a reading that is too high.) Test it in the store to be sure it's easy to use. Note that the American Heart Association doesn't recommend wrist or finger home blood pressure monitors, as they are not as reliable. For a comprehensive list of approved devices, see the website of the nonprofit Dabl Educational Trust (www.dableducational.org/sphygmomanometers.html). The Omron brand is highly rated by *Consumer Reports*.

Around-the-clock monitoring

Instead of asking you to invest in a home blood pressure monitoring unit, your doctor may send you home with a device that automatically takes your blood pressure every 15 to 30 minutes over the course of a 24-hour period and records the results. After reviewing the data, your doctor should have a better sense of your usual blood pressure. This technology, called ambulatory blood pressure monitoring, is covered by Medicare if your doctor suspects you may have white-coat or masked hypertension. But coverage by other insurers varies, so check your own policy.

Lifestyle changes to lower your blood pressure

A healthy lifestyle—which means avoiding tobacco, losing excess weight, eating nutritious foods, cutting back on salt, exercising regularly, and easing stress—is the cornerstone for preventing and treating high blood pressure.

It's hard to overstate the importance of lifestyle changes for blood pressure control. If your blood pressure is on the high side but not yet hypertensive, adopting healthier habits may be all you need to do to bring it down to a safer level. Even if you already have hypertension, it's important to make lifestyle changes, regardless of whether you are taking medications. Diligent efforts to improve your diet and fitness can add up significantly (see Table 3, below) and will very likely reduce your blood pressure numbers—possibly to the point where you don't need to pop a pill.

Even if you do need drugs to control your blood pressure, you should adopt healthy habits. The lifestyle changes described in this chapter can help medications control your blood pressure, making it possible for you to get good results with less medication. You will also reduce your risks for many chronic diseases and improve your odds of a longer, healthier life.

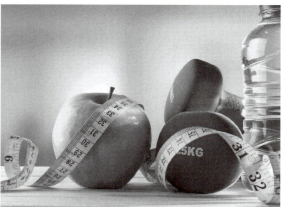

Lifestyle changes can play a key role in helping you reduce your blood pressure. In some cases, you can avoid medication altogether, or else cut a dose you're taking.

Table 3: Adding up the benefits of lifestyle changes		
LIFESTYLE CHANGE	**WHAT TO DO**	**POTENTIAL REDUCTION IN SYSTOLIC BLOOD PRESSURE IN PEOPLE WITH HIGH BLOOD PRESSURE**
Lose weight	Reach and maintain a normal body mass index.	5–20 mm Hg for every 22 pounds lost (although this varies with the individual and tends to be more in the range of 1 mm Hg for every 1–2 pounds lost)
Adopt the DASH diet	Eat plenty of fruits and vegetables, choose low-fat dairy products, and reduce total fat consumption.	11 mm Hg
Reduce salt	Cut sodium by about 1,000 mg per day.	5–6 mm Hg
Increase potassium	Aim for 3,500 to 5,000 mg daily of potassium, preferably from food.	4–5 mm Hg
Exercise regularly	Get at least 30 minutes of moderate aerobic exercise on all or most days of the week.	4–8 mm Hg (although this varies with the individual and may be as much as 11 mm Hg)
Limit alcohol	Have no more than two drinks per day if you're male, or one drink per day if you're female.	4 mm Hg
Quit smoking	There is no safe amount of cigarette smoking; if you smoke, try to quit.	2–8 mm Hg*

Source: American College of Cardiology and American Heart Association, 2017 Guideline for the Prevention, Detection, Evaluation, and Management of High Blood Pressure in Adults.
*Estimate based on clinical experience.

▶ **Tips for quitting smoking**

- ✔ **Get ready.** Set a quit date; get rid of all cigarettes and tobacco products from your home, office, and car; don't let people smoke around you; and once you quit, don't smoke—not even a puff!

- ✔ **Find support and encouragement.** Tell everyone you are going to quit and ask them not to smoke around you; talk to your health care provider; and get individual, group, or telephone counseling. Spouses, friends, co-workers, and other direct contacts have a huge influence on your odds of successfully kicking the habit. Once one person stops, others around the quitter have a better chance of quitting, too. Sometimes it helps to quit with a friend or family member so that you can support each other through the process.

- ✔ **Identify and avoid your triggers.** Many smokers link having a cigarette with activities like finishing a meal or drinking coffee or alcohol. Breaking these associations is an essential part of quitting. Counseling and social support can help you identify new ways of dealing with these triggers.

- ✔ **Learn new skills and behaviors.** Try to distract yourself by taking a walk or getting busy with a hobby or task; reduce your stress by exercising or taking a hot bath; plan something enjoyable to do each day; drink a lot of water and other nonalcoholic fluids.

Quit smoking

When it comes to blood pressure, tobacco packs a devastating wallop. Whether you smoke, chew, or vape, nicotine constricts small blood vessels, forcing the heart to work harder to circulate blood. As a result, the heart speeds up and blood pressure rises. Nicotine also interferes with some blood pressure drugs, most notably beta blockers.

When researchers tested blood pressure while people smoked, they discovered that within five minutes of lighting up, the subjects' systolic pressures rose dramatically—on average, more than 20 mm Hg—before gradually declining to their original levels over the next 30 minutes. This means the typical smoker's blood pressure soars many times throughout the day. Like people with labile hypertension (in which blood pressure may jump frequently in response to daily stresses), smokers may suffer "part-time" hyperten-

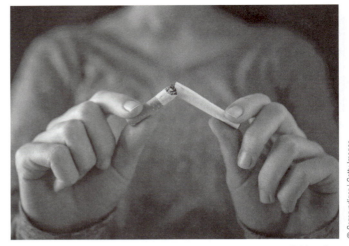

Whether you smoke, chew, or vape, nicotine constricts small blood vessels, forcing the heart to work harder. As a result, the heart speeds up and blood pressure rises for roughly 30 minutes.

sion. For example, smokers with a reading of less than 130/80 mm Hg may actually have Stage 1 hypertension every time they puff a cigarette.

Do you need more incentive to quit? The chemicals in tobacco smoke raise heart disease risk in other ways, too. They can reduce the body's oxygen supply, lower levels of HDL (good) cholesterol, and make blood platelets more likely to stick together and form clots that can trigger a heart attack.

Quitting is tough because smoking is psychologically and physically addictive. Many people make several attempts before successfully quitting, so don't give up if your first few tries don't work. Smoking cessation programs primarily address the psychological facets of addiction by helping participants change ingrained behaviors (see "Tips for quitting smoking," above left). Nicotine replacement systems—such as patches, chewing gum, and nasal sprays—target physical craving by delivering the addictive substance in another form, allowing the user to taper off gradually and minimizing withdrawal symptoms. According to the American Lung Association, combining nicotine replacement with participation in a smoking cessation program doubles your chances of successfully quitting.

Quitting offers enormous benefits. Within hours of stopping smoking, your heart rate and blood pressure decrease. Within a year of quitting, your heart disease risk is cut in half. Within 15 years of giving up smoking, your risk of heart disease is close to that of a nonsmoker.

Attain a healthy weight

Being overweight can not only raise your blood pressure, but also increase your risk for diabetes, arthritis, sleep apnea, and some cancers. Achieving and maintaining a healthy weight is an important step in fighting these and many other illnesses. Systolic and diastolic blood pressures drop an average of 1 mm Hg for every one to two pounds of weight lost, although the actual amount varies widely from person to person. A panel of experts concluded that for every 22 pounds a person loses, he or she may be able to reduce systolic blood pressure by 5 to 20 mm Hg—enough to make a real difference. Even a loss of 10 pounds can help many people.

What's a healthy weight for you? To find out, calculate your body mass index (BMI), which takes both your height and weight into consideration, at www.health.harvard.edu/BMI. A BMI of 25 to 29.9 indicates that you are overweight, while a BMI of 30 or above designates obesity.

Another thing to keep in mind is that it's not weight alone that matters, but also where you carry your extra weight. People with excess fat in the abdominal area (see Figure 6, below right) are at greater risk not only for high blood pressure, but also for high cholesterol and diabetes. So if your BMI is 25 or more, and especially if you have accumulated abdominal fat, losing weight and some of that abdominal fat can improve your health. The fat stored around your organs (visceral fat) is easier to shed than fat stored underneath the skin (subcutaneous fat).

People with high blood pressure who are more than 10% over their ideal weight may be able to reduce their blood pressure by weight loss alone (see "Tips for losing weight," page 27). For people who are very overweight or obese, weight-loss surgery lowers blood pressure and improves many other factors that raise heart disease risk. The Harvard Special Health Report *Lose Weight and Keep It Off* includes comprehensive information about these procedures and other weight-loss strategies (see "Resources," page 52).

Eat right

Even if you don't need to lose weight, eating the right foods can make a difference when it comes to fighting hypertension. Several diet plans, described below, have proved helpful for a variety of reasons. In particular, they offer lean, minimally processed foods that are packed with nutrients but not with calories. They are also naturally lower in sodium. (For more help on reducing sodium, see the Special Section, "Conquering your salt habit," beginning on page 36.)

The DASH diet

DASH stands for Dietary Approaches to Stop Hypertension, a diet developed by nutritionists to lower blood pressure. Put to the test in two large clinical trials—the first described in *The New England Journal of Medicine* in 1997—the DASH diet passed with flying colors. For many people who follow it, the diet is enough to keep

Figure 6: Check your BMI and your belly

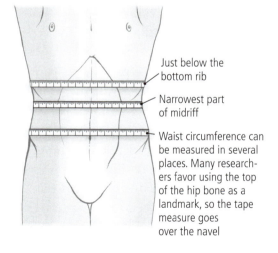

BMI categories:
- Underweight = less than 18.5
- Normal weight = 18.5–24.9
- Overweight = 25–29.9
- Obesity = 30 or greater

Waist circumference associated with increased health risks:

For men: More than 40 inches (102 cm)
For women: More than 35 inches (88 cm)

© Jason Laramie

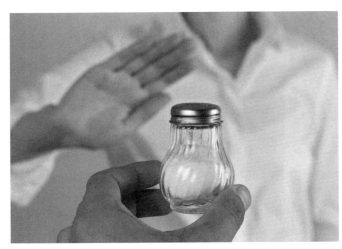

The DASH diet was developed to reduce blood pressure. It is lower in salt than a standard diet and higher in potassium and heart-healthy fruits and vegetables, all of which help lower blood pressure.

blood pressure in the normal range without medicine.

Key features of the DASH diet include plenty of fruits, vegetables, and whole grains; several servings daily of low-fat dairy products; some fish, poultry, dried beans, nuts, and seeds; and minimal red meat, sweets, and sugar-laden beverages. This mix of foods provides ample calcium, potassium, magnesium, vitamins, and fiber while limiting saturated fat, cholesterol, and sodium (see Table 4, page 28). (Although canned beans are convenient, they often contain too much salt, even if you drain and rinse them. So it's best to buy dried beans, which can be soaked overnight to speed up cooking.)

Researchers do not attribute the blood pressure reductions of the DASH trial to any single nutrient. Compared with the typical American diet, the DASH eating plan has a relatively higher calcium content and less sodium, total fat, saturated fat, and cholesterol. It also has 173% more magnesium, 150% more potassium, 240% more fiber, and 30% more protein.

In the original DASH study, 459 volunteers were randomly assigned one of three diets:
- The first was based on what most Americans eat, including daily servings of meat, chicken, or fish, regular-fat dairy products, and snacks and sweets, with 37% of calories from fat.
- The second was a similar regimen, but with fruits and vegetables added.
- The third was the DASH diet, which includes plenty of fruits and vegetables, whole grains, low-fat or nonfat dairy products, and small amounts of meat, fish, poultry, and nuts, with 27% of calories from fat.

After following the DASH plan for eight weeks, participants with high blood pressure experienced average reductions of 11.4 mm Hg in systolic pressure and 5.5 mm Hg in diastolic pressure. These results are comparable to the effects of some drugs. Even participants with borderline high blood pressure experienced improvements, suggesting that the DASH diet might keep some people from developing hypertension in the first place.

The second diet, which was higher in fats but rich in fruits and vegetables, also lowered blood pressure in all participants (both with and without high blood pressure) by 2.8 mm Hg systolic pressure and 1.1 mm Hg diastolic pressure. All reductions occurred without people changing their salt intake, alcohol consumption, or weight—factors known to influence blood pressure.

Participants following the standard American diet saw no improvements.

A follow-up analysis of the trial's results found that the DASH diet reduced blood pressure in virtually all groups tested regardless of such factors as age, sex, race, and hypertension status. Its effects were most pronounced, though, in African Americans and people with high blood pressure. In fact, the results were so promising that the federal guidelines recommend that all Americans—not just those with high blood pressure—follow the DASH diet.

A follow-up study, the DASH-Sodium trial, compared a typical American diet (the control diet) with the DASH diet at different sodium levels (3,300, 2,400, or 1,500 mg per day). People with high blood pressure who ate the DASH diet at the lowest sodium level had an average systolic pressure reading 11.5 mm Hg lower than participants eating the control diet at the highest sodium level (see "A low-salt DASH diet helps prevent age-related blood pressure rise," page 29).

Still more support for the DASH diet came from an assessment from the Harvard-based Nurses' Health Study. Among nearly 90,000 female nurses whose diets, other habits, and health were followed for 24 years, those whose eating patterns most closely resembled the DASH diet had fewer heart attacks and strokes and were less likely to have died of heart disease compared with women reporting average American diets. Other research suggests that combining a structured weight-loss program with the DASH diet can lower your blood pressure even more than the DASH diet alone.

Beyond DASH: OmniHeart

The OmniHeart study, which tested three different diets, took DASH a step further by replacing some of its carbohydrates with unsaturated fat or protein. Investigators wanted to assess the impact not only on blood pressure, but also on cholesterol.

In the study, researchers from Harvard and other medical institutions asked 164 people with prehypertension or Stage 1 hypertension (according to the 2017 reclassification, this would be Stage 1 and Stage 2, respectively) to follow three different diets in random sequence. One diet was high in carbohydrates, another high in protein, and the third high in unsaturated fat. All of the diets were healthy in that they included lots of fruits, vegetables, and whole grains. Meats were limited to lean cuts and skinless poultry. Dairy products were nonfat or low-fat.

The results of the OmniHeart trial, published in *The Journal of the American Medical Association*, were striking. When the participants' blood pressure and cholesterol levels were tested after six weeks on each diet, the researchers found that all three diets lowered blood pressure, improved cholesterol profiles, and lowered risk of heart disease. But the high-protein diet

Tips for losing weight

Weight loss comes down to the simple fact that you have to burn off more calories than you consume. What's not so easy is actually doing that over the long haul. Your body has evolved to protect you against famine and starvation and will fight against sustained weight loss, either by slowing metabolism or by pumping up hunger hormones to get you to eat more once you go off a weight-loss diet. Here are some strategies to help you fight back.

Boost your routine, everyday activity. Exercise is one obvious way to burn off calories, and it has countless benefits for your overall health. Weight loss may even be one of them. But all too often, any potential weight loss is offset by the extra calories you wolf down afterward in order to replenish your energy. So yes, by all means, exercise. But also try to increase your everyday activity—gardening, walking, hanging laundry up to dry, pacing while talking on the phone, climbing stairs instead of taking the elevator. In some studies, the sole difference between lean and obese people was the amount of everyday activity in their lives.

Skip the sipped calories. Your body needs plenty of fluids, but it pays to be selective when pouring. Soda, lattes, sports drinks, energy drinks, and even fruit juices are all packed with unnecessary calories—and it's surprising how quickly they all add up. Worse, your body doesn't seem to account for liquid calories the same way it registers solid calories, so you can keep right on chugging them before your internal satiety mechanisms tell you to stop. Instead, try unsweetened coffee or tea, or flavor your own sparkling water with a slice of lemon or lime, a sprig of fresh mint, a few raspberries, or an ounce or two of 100% fruit juice.

Eat more whole foods. Processed foods, particularly those containing refined carbohydrates and added sugars—think chips, cookies, candy, and the like—can pack a lot of calories into a small amount of food that is quickly digested and soon leaves you hungry again. If your road to weight loss is simply to restrict these foods, you will soon feel deprived and start eating more. But if you substitute unprocessed foods—think fruits, vegetables, and whole grains—you can eat a great quantity of food and fill yourself up on meals that take a long time to digest. You'll feel fuller longer. Plus, whole foods have more vitamins, minerals, and fiber—and because they're much lower in sodium, they're better for your blood pressure, too.

Find healthier snacks. Snack time is many people's downfall. Don't let it be yours. Most nutritionists today support the idea of snacking during the day to keep your blood sugar levels steady, but do it wisely. For example, carrot sticks are sweet and crunchy and make a fine substitute for potato chips or crackers (and without the salt in crackers and chips). Air-popped popcorn also makes a good, low-calorie snack, provided you skip the butter. (It doesn't have to taste bland. Instead of adding butter and salt, try seasoning it with your favorite spices.) Snacks that provide some healthy fat and some protein seem to be particularly satisfying, so try a dollop of sunflower seed butter on apple slices. Unsalted nuts are another filling, healthy snack.

Table 4: The DASH eating plan

The DASH eating plan shown below is based on 2,000 calories a day. The number of daily servings in a food group may vary from those listed depending on your caloric needs. To learn more about the DASH diet, visit www.health.harvard.edu/dash-diet.

FOOD GROUP	EXAMPLES	SERVINGS
Grains and grain products	1 slice bread 1 cup ready-to-eat cereal* ½ cup cooked rice, pasta, or cereal	7–8 per day
Vegetables	1 cup raw leafy vegetable ½ cup cooked vegetable 6 ounces vegetable juice	4–5 per day
Fruits	1 medium fruit ¼ cup dried fruit ½ cup fresh, frozen, or canned fruit 6 ounces fruit juice	4–5 per day
Low-fat or fat-free dairy foods	8 ounces milk 1 cup yogurt 1½ ounces cheese	2–3 per day
Lean meats, poultry, and fish	3 ounces cooked lean meats, skinless poultry, or fish	2 or less per day
Nuts, seeds, and beans	½ cup or 1½ ounces nuts 1 tablespoon or ½ ounce seeds ½ cup cooked dry beans	4–5 per week
Fats and oils**	1 teaspoon soft margarine 1 tablespoon low-fat mayonnaise 2 tablespoons light salad dressing 1 teaspoon vegetable oil	2–3 per day
Sweets	1 tablespoon sugar 1 tablespoon jelly or jam ½ ounce jelly beans 8 ounces lemonade	5 per week

*Serving sizes vary between ½ cup and 1¼ cups. Check the product's nutrition label.
**Fat content changes serving counts for fats and oils: for example, 1 tablespoon of regular salad dressing equals 1 serving; 1 tablespoon of a low-fat dressing equals ½ serving; 1 tablespoon of a fat-free dressing equals 0 servings.

LDL cholesterol by 12 milligrams per deciliter (mg/dL), but also slightly lowered beneficial HDL cholesterol.

High–unsaturated fat diet. The diet high in unsaturated fats, dubbed the UNSAT diet, outperformed the high-carb DASH-like diet. It lowered blood pressure, increased HDL cholesterol, and lowered triglycerides (another fat that circulates in the blood and correlates with heart disease). Results showed that eating lots of unsaturated fats—primarily monounsaturated fats from vegetable oils and nuts—lowered blood pressure in people with hypertension 3 points more than the DASH-like diet, for a total drop of 16 points.

The UNSAT diet also was the only diet that did not lower HDL cholesterol, but raised it slightly. That's good, because while there are a number of ways to lower LDL cholesterol, such as taking medication, it's more difficult to raise HDL level. HDLs, or high-density lipoprotein particles, sweep your blood clean of unhealthy fats, preventing the buildup of fatty plaque that narrows your arteries.

High-protein diet. The good news for protein lovers is that the high-protein diet also did better than the high-carb DASH-like diet. It lowered systolic blood pressure 3.5 points more than the high-carb diet in people with Stage 1 hypertension, for a total 16.5-point reduction. The high-protein diet also lowered LDL cholesterol 3 points more than the high-carb diet, but like the high-carb diet, slightly lowered healthy HDLs as well. The high-protein plan did the best of the three diets in lowering triglycerides—another good step in lowering risk of heart disease. If you decide to go a high-protein route, choose healthy protein "packages" like chicken, turkey, beans, nuts, low-fat dairy foods, and lean red meat. Loading up on bunless bacon burgers and hot dogs won't get you to your goal.

Mediterranean diet

Another similar eating style that's been shown to lower blood pressure (as well as promote weight loss and lower heart disease risk) is a cuisine based on the traditional diets of people living in Greece, Italy, and other Mediterranean countries. In general, a Mediterranean-type diet is low in saturated fat and high in fiber. Fruits, vegetables, grains, beans, nuts, and seeds are eaten daily and make up about half of the diet. Fat,

and the high–unsaturated fat diet both delivered even greater health benefits than the high-carbohydrate DASH-like diet did by improving blood pressure and cholesterol levels even more. Here are the findings:

High-carb diet. The high-carb DASH-like diet lowered systolic blood pressure by 13 points in people with Stage 1 hypertension and 7 points in those with prehypertension. The high-carb diet also lowered harmful much of it from olive oil, may account for up to 40% of daily calories. Cheese or yogurt is usually eaten each day, along with a serving of fish, poultry, or eggs, and red meat on occasion. Small amounts of red wine are typically taken with meals, and regular physical activity is a part of daily life.

A large Spanish study of 7,500 people at risk of heart disease, called PREDIMED, compared three diets: a reduced-fat diet, a Mediterranean diet supplemented with nuts, or a Mediterranean diet supplemented with minimally processed (extra-virgin) olive oil. Both forms of the Mediterranean diet lowered 24-hour ambulatory blood pressure (see "Around-the-clock monitoring," page 22) compared with the reduced-fat diet. Earlier reports from PREDIMED found that people following the two Mediterranean diets also had lower rates of heart attacks, strokes, and diabetes.

Notes on specific nutrients

Below are summaries of the current thinking on how specific nutrients—alcohol, caffeine, sugar, and certain minerals—may affect blood pressure.

Alcohol. Despite popular belief that moderate drinking is good for your heart, the evidence to support that claim is fairly weak. People who drink moderate amounts of alcohol—defined as no more than one drink a day for women or two drinks for men (see "What's a standard drink?" on page 30)—tend to have lower rates of coronary artery disease than people who avoid alcohol. But it's not clear whether their drinking habits or some other lifestyle factor is responsible for the lower risk.

What's more, heavier drinking raises the risk of high blood pressure and heart disease (see "Heavy drinking," page 15). How alcohol raises blood pressure

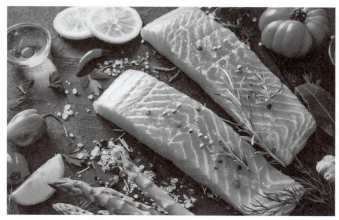

In addition to the DASH diet, a Mediterranean-style diet has been shown to lower blood pressure, promote weight loss, and lower heart disease risk.

A low-salt DASH diet helps prevent age-related blood pressure rise

A low-sodium DASH diet may prevent or reverse the typical rise in blood pressure that occurs as people grow older, according to findings from the DASH-Sodium trial. The study included just over 400 people, with roughly half following a typical American diet (the control group) and half following the DASH diet for three months. During that time, both groups ate three versions of their assigned diet with different sodium levels: high (3,500 mg), intermediate (2,300 mg), and low (1,200 mg) for a month each. Researchers also divided the volunteers into four subgroups according to age; each subgroup is represented by a single point in the graph at right.

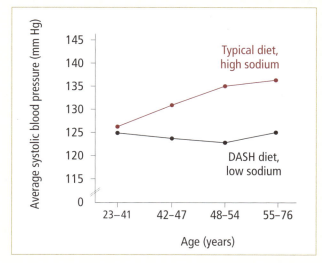

The red line shows the typical rise in average systolic blood pressure over time on a standard diet, as indicated by the four control groups at the end of their high-sodium phase. The values for those in the oldest age group rose to a level that would be categorized as Stage 1 hypertension under the current guidelines. By contrast, the black line shows the DASH groups at the end of their low-sodium phase. On the low-sodium DASH diet, average systolic blood pressures measured around 125 mm Hg, even in the oldest age group.

Source: New England Journal of Medicine (2010), Vol. 362, pp. 2102–12.

Table 5: Selected potassium-rich foods

FOOD	POTASSIUM (MG)
Sweet potato, baked, 1 medium	694
Baked potato, 1 medium, without skin	610
Yogurt, plain, low-fat, 8 ounces	531
White beans, cooked, ½ cup	502
Halibut, cooked, 3 ounces	490
Soybeans, green, cooked (edamame), ½ cup	485
Yellowfin tuna, cooked, 3 ounces	484
Banana, 1 medium	422
Spinach, cooked, ½ cup	419
Milk, nonfat, 1 cup	382
Apricots, dried, ¼ cup	378
Cantaloupe, ¼ medium	368
Orange juice, ¾ cup	355
Raisins, 1 small box (1.5 ounces)	322
Tomato, 1 medium	292
Grapes, 1 cup	176

Source: U.S. Department of Agriculture National Nutrient Database.

Table 6: Selected calcium-rich foods

FOOD	CALCIUM (MG)
Yogurt, plain, low-fat, 8 ounces	415
Collards, frozen, cooked, 1 cup	357
Rhubarb, frozen, cooked, 1 cup	348
Yogurt, fruit, low-fat, 8 ounces	345
Sardines, canned, with bones, 3 ounces	325
Milk, skim or fat-free, 1 cup	306
Spinach,* frozen, cooked, 1 cup	291
Milk, 1% milkfat, 1 cup	290
Cheese, mozzarella, 1 ounce	207
Salmon, canned, with bones, 3 ounces	181
Kale, frozen, cooked, 1 cup	179
Tofu,** firm, 4 ounces	163
Bok choy, fresh, cooked, 1 cup	158

*Spinach contains oxalic acid, which interferes with calcium absorption.
**Tofu made with calcium sulfate.
Source: U.S. Department of Agriculture National Nutrient Database.

What's a standard drink?

- 1½ ounces (a jigger) of 80-proof liquor (bourbon, brandy, gin, rum, scotch, tequila, vodka, or whiskey)
- 2–3 ounces of liqueur with fruit, coffee, chocolate, or other flavoring (cordials)
- 3–4 ounces of fortified wine (sherry, port, marsala, or Madeira)
- 5 ounces of table wine
- 12 ounces of regular or light beer

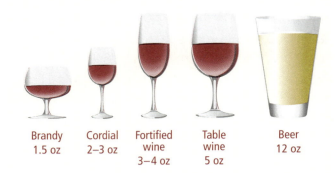

Brandy 1.5 oz | Cordial 2–3 oz | Fortified wine 3–4 oz | Table wine 5 oz | Beer 12 oz

is unknown, but it appears that once you go past two drinks per day, the more you drink, the higher your blood pressure. This effect becomes more pronounced as you age and occurs regardless of what type of alcohol you drink. As noted earlier, heavy drinking also interferes with blood pressure medication and may boost the risk of stroke and heart failure.

Drinking has dietary drawbacks, too. For people battling their weight, alcohol adds "empty" calories with no nutritional value. Alcohol has 7 calories per gram, compared with 4 calories per gram for carbohydrates—or 0 for water. A bottle of beer contains 146 calories (100 calories if it's light beer), and a glass of wine has 123 calories. Some mixed drinks add fat and cholesterol, too. Eggnog with brandy, for example, serves up 288 calories with 6 grams of saturated fat, 11 grams of total fat, and 84 mg of cholesterol. Other mixed drinks, such as a Scotch and soda or a whiskey with ginger ale, are better choices from a caloric perspective.

In addition to watching your alcohol consumption, pay attention to sodium when you consume certain drinks. A Bloody Mary contains a tremendous amount of sodium because of the tomato juice.

Caffeine. Most experts believe that caffeine may raise blood pressure in people who are unaccustomed to consuming it, but not in regular users. Unless you are consuming large amounts of caffeine, its effect on your blood pressure is likely to be minimal. The current blood pressure guidelines recommend limiting caffeine to 300 milligrams (mg) per day (about the amount in three cups of regular coffee).

Sugar. Drinking less soda and other sugar-sweetened beverages may help lower blood pressure. People with high blood pressure who cut one sugary drink per day (about 12 ounces) from their diets lowered their blood pressure by about 1.8/1.1 mm Hg, one study found. (Americans drink an average of 2.3 sugar-sweetened beverages, or about 28 ounces, a day.)

Other research has found links between a high intake of fructose (a form of sugar that makes up 50% or more of table sugar and the high-fructose corn syrup often used in soft drinks and processed foods) and a higher risk of developing hypertension. Don't let the fructose warnings scare you away from eating fruit—you can't get harmful levels of it by eating fresh fruit—but there can be a great deal of fructose in processed foods. Although further research is needed to verify these findings, it's still a good idea to steer clear of sugary foods and beverages because they provide zero nutrients but lots of calories. If nothing else, those calories can contribute to weight gain, which can also raise blood pressure.

Potassium. People with diets high in potassium have lower blood pressure than those with potassium-poor diets. Potassium helps reduce blood pressure because it helps the body get rid of excess sodium and relaxes blood vessels. Plenty of heart-healthy foods contain potassium—most notably, vegetables, legumes, and fruits (see Table 5, page 30). These foods also tend to be lower in sodium, providing a double benefit when it comes to lowering blood pressure. (For more about the relationship between sodium and potassium, see the Special Section, "Conquering your salt habit," page 36.)

Federal guidelines recommend 4,700 mg of potassium per day for adults—a level that was easily attainable in the days of our hunter-gatherer ancestors. Unfortunately, most Americans today fall far short. In

A warning on potassium pills and salt substitutes

Although potassium is essential—and most Americans get way too little of it in their diets—potassium supplements and potassium-based salt substitutes are potentially risky if you're taking certain heart drugs or have impaired kidney function.

Many medications, especially blood pressure drugs, can affect your potassium level. For example, ACE inhibitors, such as lisinopril (Prinvil, Zestril) or ramipril (Altace), may raise potassium levels. So can common painkillers such as ibuprofen (Advil, Motrin) or naproxen (Aleve).

Trickiest is the class of blood pressure medications known as diuretics. Some of these drugs, such as hydrochlorothiazide (Microzide) or furosemide (Lasix), tend to *lower* potassium levels, while others—the so-called potassium-sparing diuretics, such as spironolactone (Aldactone)—have the opposite effect, *raising* potassium.

Keeping your blood potassium level in the correct range is important, because this mineral also plays a key role in the function of nerves and muscles, including heart muscle. Your kidneys help regulate potassium levels in your blood. But age, diabetes, heart failure, and certain other conditions may impair kidney function. As a result, potassium levels can rise to high levels, and, in extreme cases, lead to dangerous heart rhythm problems and even cardiac arrest. Very low potassium levels are also dangerous.

Here's how to stay in the right range:

- **If you have normal kidney function**, keeping track of your potassium levels is not a serious concern.

- **If you have kidney disease or take a drug that raises potassium levels**, be careful to monitor your potassium. Some people trying to curb their sodium intake use potassium-based salt substitutes. But you should be aware that a mere one-quarter teaspoon of one brand contains about 800 mg of potassium (out of a recommended 4,700 mg per day). If you take an ACE inhibitor, painkillers, or a potassium-sparing diuretic, you should avoid salt substitutes and limit high-potassium foods.

- **If you take a diuretic that lowers your potassium level**, increase the potassium in your diet or take a supplement. Your doctor may prescribe extended-release potassium tablets, which contain 600 to 750 mg of the mineral.

If you take any diuretic or ACE inhibitor, ask your doctor whether you need periodic testing of your potassium and kidney function, to be on the safe side.

the DASH diet studies, people following the diet ate an average of 8.5 servings of fruits and vegetables a day—and consumed 4,100 mg of potassium. Those on the standard American diet ate only 3.5 daily servings of fruits and vegetables, providing just 1,700 mg of daily potassium.

That said, you should get your potassium from natural foods rather than from pills. In fact, experts warn people taking blood pressure drugs not to use potassium supplements or potassium-based salt substitutes unless your doctor prescribes them, because they could upset the potassium balance in your body and put you at risk for too high or too low levels of the mineral (see "A warning on potassium pills and salt substitutes," page 31).

Calcium. Calcium is important for healthy blood pressure because it helps blood vessels tighten and relax when they need to. The best evidence for calcium's power to lower blood pressure comes from the success of the DASH diet, which includes two servings of low-fat dairy products per day (see Table 6, page 30, for other good sources).

Low calcium intake may contribute to high blood pressure, perhaps because it predisposes your body to retain sodium, which raises blood pressure. But efforts to control blood pressure with calcium supplements have had mixed results. For most people, supplements have no effect or reduce blood pressure only slightly—by an average of 1 to 2 mm Hg in systolic readings. However, many Americans don't get recommended amounts of calcium in their diets, so many doctors recommend supplements. Adults ages 19 to 50 should get 1,000 mg daily, and people ages 51 and older should get 1,200 mg a day.

Magnesium. Like calcium, this mineral helps blood vessels tighten and relax when they need to. It also helps regulate blood sugar and nerve function. Dietary surveys show that most people in the United States—especially men over age 70—don't get the recommended amount of magnesium from

> **ASK THE DOCTOR**
>
> **Q** *Can I lift heavy weights if I have high blood pressure?*
>
> **A** In the past, doctors were hesitant to recommend any type of strength training for people with high blood pressure, because this type of exercise causes a short-term spike in blood pressure. But information from the American Heart Association suggests that moderate, comfortable resistance exercises are safe and beneficial for general health, even if they don't do anything to improve your blood pressure readings.
>
> According to the Physical Activity Guidelines for Americans from the U.S. Department of Health and Human Services, strength training should be performed two or three days per week. But don't overdo it. We're talking about maintaining muscle tone, not becoming a body builder. "Moderate" resistance exercises mean starting with resistance bands, small hand weights, or weight machines. Generally speaking, you should aim to perform one or two sets of eight to 12 repetitions of each exercise, using a weight that's challenging but manageable.
>
> And make sure to breathe! Blood pressure can soar to dangerous levels if you hold your breath while performing strength exercises—or for that matter, lifting heavy boxes or furniture. That sudden rise could be enough to burst a plaque in one of your arteries, causing a stroke or heart attack. So it's important to exhale as you lift, push, or pull; inhale as you release. If you find yourself "grunting" or getting stuck in the middle of a lift, you're using too much weight. Decrease the amount of weight to stay in a safe zone.

Table 7: Selected magnesium-rich foods

FOOD	MAGNESIUM (MG)
Almonds, dry-roasted, 1 ounce	80
Spinach, boiled, ½ cup	78
Peanuts, oil-roasted, ¼ cup	63
Cereal, shredded wheat, 2 large biscuits	61
Soymilk, plain or vanilla, 1 cup	61
Black beans, cooked, ½ cup	60
Peanut butter, smooth, 2 tablespoons	49
Bread, whole-wheat, 2 slices	46
Avocado, cubed, 1 cup	44
Rice, brown, cooked, ½ cup	42
Yogurt, plain, low-fat, 8 ounces	42

Source: Office of Dietary Supplements, National Institutes of Health.

the foods they eat. Men should get 420 mg of magnesium a day and women should consume 320 mg daily (see Table 7, page 32).

Some people with certain medical problems—such as Crohn's disease, celiac disease, or poorly controlled type 2 diabetes—may be more likely than others to have lower magnesium levels. In addition, two widely used types of drugs can deplete magnesium levels. Long-term use of heartburn drugs known as proton-pump inhibitors—including omeprazole (Prilosec) and lansoprazole (Prevacid)—may interfere with magnesium absorption. Diuretics such as hydrochlorothiazide (Microzide) and furosemide (Lasix), which are prescribed to treat high blood pressure, cause magnesium to be flushed out in the urine.

It's possible—but far from proven—that certain people with high blood pressure might benefit from magnesium supplements. Don't take them without consulting your doctor first. There are no known adverse affects of magnesium intake from food. But high doses from supplements or magnesium-containing drugs (for example, laxatives like Phillips' Milk of Magnesia) may cause diarrhea.

Be active

Not only does regular exercise help prevent high blood pressure, but it's also a proven way to lower high blood pressure in people who have it already. The more physically active you are, the lower your risk.

The American College of Sports Medicine reviewed 40 studies on the effect of exercise on blood pressure. With regular aerobic exercise, participants were able to reduce their systolic and diastolic pressures by an average of 11 and 9 mm Hg, respectively. Although many studies focused on high-intensity exercises like running, several evaluated the impact of moderate activities such as walking. Surprisingly, moderate-intensity training provided the same or even better blood pressure benefits. And, in some trials, blood pressure dropped enough for people to reduce their medications.

Need more reasons to get up and moving? Exercise reduces cholesterol, helps prevent plaque buildup in the arteries, and makes unwanted clots less likely. It helps strengthen muscles and bones, helps control weight, and even improves mood and mental functioning. For blood pressure reduction, aerobic activity is the type of exercise you want. Strength training exercises, such as lifting weights and doing resistance-band workouts, are great for your overall health, but will temporarily boost blood pressure. (For more detail, see "Ask the Doctor," page 32.) Note that a related activity—shoveling snow—can also cause blood pressure to rise. Doing such intense exercise in cold temperatures (which can constrict arteries) makes shoveling snow uniquely dangerous for people with high blood pressure, so it should be avoided.

The Physical Activity Guidelines for Americans recommend that adults get two hours and 30 minutes of moderate-intensity aerobic exercise a week. Alternatively, you can substitute one hour and 15 minutes of vigorous exercise or an equivalent combination of the two. You can break up your total exercise time into smaller segments, but make sure each period of exercise lasts for at least 10 minutes. Increasing your exercise to five hours of moderate-intensity exercise per week (or two hours and 30 minutes of vigorous exercise) yields even greater health rewards. But it's important to start any exercise program slowly and to gradually build up the intensity level and length of sessions. People with heart disease or other health problems should consult their doctors before starting an exercise program.

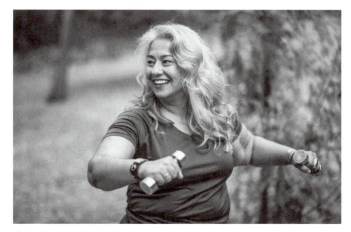

If you have high blood pressure, regular exercise may enable you to reduce your medication. Even moderate activity such as walking pays off. Aim for 30 minutes a day most days of the week.

Meditation and a relaxation technique to lower blood pressure

Several practices that help calm the mind can also lower blood pressure. All are types of meditation, which use different methods to reach a state sometimes described as "thoughtful awareness" or "restful alertness."

But while researchers are now beginning to better understand how these mental changes affect the cardiovascular system, studying meditation has proved somewhat challenging. For one thing, some studies don't include a good control treatment to compare with meditation. Second, the people most likely to volunteer for a meditation study are often already sold on meditation's benefits and so are more likely to report positive effects.

Still, a number of well-designed studies show that meditation can modestly lower blood pressure, according to an American Heart Association scientific statement published in the journal *Hypertension*.

To get a sense of mindfulness meditation, you can try one of the guided recordings by Dr. Ronald Siegel, an assistant clinical professor of psychology at Harvard Medical School. They are available for free at www.mindfulness-solution.com. Some people find that learning mindfulness techniques and practicing them with a group is especially helpful. Mindfulness-based stress reduction training, developed by Dr. Jon Kabat-Zinn at the University of Massachusetts Medical School in Worcester, Mass., is now widely available in cities throughout the United States.

A related technique, designed to evoke the so-called relaxation response, was developed by Dr. Herbert Benson, director emeritus of the Harvard-affiliated Benson-Henry Institute for Mind Body Medicine. The relaxation response is the opposite of the stress-induced fight-or-flight response. This self-induced quieting of brain activity has aspects of both transcendental meditation and mindfulness meditation.

Dr. Benson's research has found that this technique can help with high blood pressure and other disorders caused or made worse by stress. In one study, elderly people with hard-to-treat isolated systolic hypertension who underwent relaxation response training were more likely to be able to control their blood pressure to the point where they could eliminate their blood pressure medications (see "Can stress reduction lower your need for medication?" on page 50). Further research revealed that when blood pressure falls during the relaxation response, genes that promote inflammation and blood vessel constriction become less active, whereas genes involved in widening blood vessels become more active.

This benefit also may be mediated by nitric oxide, a molecule made in the body that (among other things) helps relax and widen blood vessels, keeping blood pressure under control. A small study found that people who practiced the relaxation response for eight weeks had higher levels of nitric oxide in their breath, while a control group showed no such change.

Dr. Benson recommends practicing the relaxation response twice a day, for 10 to 20 minutes, similar to what other meditation experts recommend. Here's how to do it.

- Sit in a quiet place with your eyes closed.
- Relax your muscles and silently repeat a word, phrase, sound, or short prayer of your choosing over and over.
- When stray thoughts interfere (as they will), let them come and go and return to your word, phrase, or sound.

For additional ideas, see "Quick stress-relief exercises" on page 35.

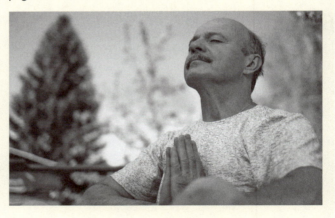

Stress less

Even though it's vital to survival, stress has a bad reputation. When you perceive stress, your sympathetic nervous system triggers the fight-or-flight response to prepare your body for action. A release of hormones quickens your heart rate and breathing, and extra blood is pumped to your muscles and organs to provide them with a burst of energy. Stress keeps drivers alert, helps students excel, and spurs competitors to win. But ongoing stress has harmful long-term effects, including raising your blood pressure.

Your fight-or-flight reaction may be stimulated in situations where you perceive a lack of control, such as in the workplace. A number of studies examining work-related stress have found an association between high stress on the job and increased blood pressure at

Quick stress-relief exercises

When you've got one minute. Place your hand just beneath your navel so you can feel the gentle rise and fall of your belly as you breathe. Breathe in. Pause for a count of three. Breathe out. Pause for a count of three. Continue to breathe deeply for one minute, pausing for a count of three after each inhalation and exhalation.

When you've got three minutes. While sitting down, take a break from whatever you're doing and check your body for tension. Relax your facial muscles and allow your jaw to fall open slightly. Let your shoulders drop. Let your arms fall to your sides. Allow your hands to loosen so that there are spaces between your fingers. Uncross your legs or ankles. Feel your thighs sink into your chair, letting your legs fall comfortably apart. Feel your shins and calves become heavier and your feet grow roots into the floor. Now breathe in slowly and breathe out slowly. Each time you breathe out, try to relax even more.

When you've got 10 minutes. Try imagery. Start by sitting comfortably in a quiet room. Breathe deeply and evenly for a few minutes. Now picture yourself in a special place. Choose an image that conjures up good memories. What do you smell—the heavy scent of roses on a hot day, crisp fall air, the aroma of baking bread? What do you hear? Drink in the colors and shapes that surround you. Focus on sensory pleasures: the swoosh of a gentle wind, the soft cool grass tickling your feet. Passively observe intrusive thoughts and then gently disengage from them to return to the world you've created.

---

work, at home, and during sleep. One study also noted that feeling overcommitted and poorly rewarded for effort at work may be related to blood pressure both in and outside of the workplace.

Social relationships play an important role in your body's response to stress. Family members and friends often provide emotional support and can help mitigate stressful situations. But relationships are a source of conflict at times. A strained marriage, for example, may produce increases in blood pressure. A recent study suggests that difficult interactions with your spouse or partner can elevate blood pressure and heart rate, essentially mimicking a fight-or-flight response.

Of course, stressful events are often not within your control. But developing effective coping mechanisms can help. If you are often tense, try the following stress-reduction strategies.

Get enough sleep. Lack of sound sleep can affect your mood, mental alertness, energy level, and physical health.

Exercise. Physical activity alleviates stress and reduces your risk of becoming depressed.

Learn relaxation techniques. Meditation, progressive muscle relaxation, guided imagery, deep breathing exercises, and yoga are the mainstays of stress relief. Your local hospital or community center may offer meditation or yoga classes, or you can learn about these techniques from books or videos. (See also "Meditation and a relaxation technique to lower blood pressure," page 34, and "Quick stress-relief exercises," above.)

Strengthen your social network. Studies show that social ties significantly protect health and well-being in multiple ways. Try to connect with others by taking a class, joining an organization, or participating in a support group.

Learn time-management skills. These skills can help you juggle work and family demands.

Confront stressful situations head-on. Don't let stressful situations fester. Hold family problem-solving sessions and use negotiation skills at work.

Nurture yourself. Treat yourself to a massage. Truly savor an experience: eat slowly, focusing on each bite of that orange, or soak up the warm rays of the sun or the scent of blooming flowers during a walk outdoors. Take a nap. Enjoy the sounds of music you find calming.

Talk to your doctor. If stress and anxiety persist, ask your doctor whether anti-anxiety medications could be helpful. ♥

SPECIAL SECTION

Conquering your salt habit

Salt—sodium chloride—is essential for survival. Your body depends on sodium to transmit nerve impulses, contract muscle fibers, and, along with potassium, to balance fluid levels in all your cells. Because the human body is so good at conserving this vital mineral, you need only a tiny amount of sodium. In fact, individuals in some populations, like the South American Yanomamo Indians, consume a mere 200 mg of sodium—about the amount in one-tenth of a teaspoon of salt—per day.

Thousands of years ago, when humans roamed the earth gathering and hunting, sodium was scarce. By contrast, potassium—found naturally in many plant-based foods—was abundant. In fact, the average diet in Paleolithic times provided roughly 16 times more potassium than sodium (see Figure 7, page 37).

Today, the average American diet contains about twice as much sodium as potassium, as a result of the high levels of sodium in processed foods (see "Where's the salt?" at right). This sodium-potassium imbalance, which is at odds with how humans evolved, is thought to be a major contributor to high blood pressure. Though it's not completely clear how potassium works, it maintains a sort of yin-yang relationship with sodium, dialing down blood pressure where sodium ratchets it up—provided there's enough potassium in the diet to have this beneficial effect.

Findings from the Trials of Hypertension Prevention study suggest that reversing the imbalance between the two minerals can help the heart and arteries. Researchers measured the amounts of sodium and potassium excreted over the course of 24 hours by nearly 3,000 volunteers. (The amount excreted is a good stand-in for the amount consumed.) The higher the ratio of sodium to potassium, the greater the chance of having a heart attack or stroke, needing bypass surgery or angioplasty, or dying of cardiovascular disease over 10 to 15 years of follow-up. To reverse the ratio, choose foods with a high proportion of potassium to sodium (see Table 8, page 39).

Where's the salt?

Salt plays many roles in food, from acting as a preservative or a binder to helping yeast rise. It is also a cheap way to make food tastier. More than 40% of the sodium Americans consume each day comes from only 10 types of food, ranked here according to sodium content and how often people eat these foods.

1. Breads and rolls
2. Pizza
3. Sandwiches
4. Cold cuts and cured meats
5. Soups
6. Burritos and tacos
7. Savory snacks (e.g., chips and pretzels)
8. Chicken
9. Cheese
10. Eggs and omelets

Source: Centers for Disease Control and Prevention.

The hazards of excess salt

When you take in more sodium than you need, your body responds by holding on to water to dilute the sodium. As a result, the amount of fluid within your blood vessels increases. That raises the pressure inside your blood vessels and makes the heart work harder. In fact, excess sodium essentially counteracts the benefits of two types of blood pressure medications—namely, diuretics and vasodilators. Diuretics help flush excess fluid and sodium from the body, while vasodilators relax blood vessel walls. A high-sodium diet, however, will cause the body to retain additional extra fluid and refill your relaxed arteries, putting you back where you started.

Dozens of studies show that blood pressure rises with higher levels of sodium in the diet, although some people are more salt-sensitive than others. A report in the journal *BMJ* underscored the health hazards of a high-sodium diet. Researchers pooled results from 13 studies that involved more than 177,000 people who were followed between 3.5 and 19 years. Higher sodium intake was linked to 23% more strokes and 14% more cases of heart disease.

But does cutting back on salt save lives? Despite some earlier skepticism, the current consensus is clearly yes. Several studies have shown that lowering dietary sodium leads to a drop in deaths from heart attacks, strokes, and other cardiovascular causes. One example comes from a study in *BMJ Open*, which relied on data from England, where the country's Food Standards Agency set sodium-reduction targets for processed foods. From 2003 to 2011, sodium consumption by British people fell 15%. Over that same time, blood pressure fell by an average of 3 points systolic and 1.4 point diastolic. Most impressively, deaths from heart attacks and strokes dropped by 40% and 42%, respectively.

A salt step-down?

In 2012, the World Health Organization recommended a dietary target of no more than 5 grams of salt (about 2,000 mg of sodium) per day. And in the United States, the Institute of Medicine has recommended that the FDA require reductions in the amount of sodium in commercially prepared food. Such a move could theoretically make a big difference, since most of the sodium in the American diet is put there by someone else—a food company, chef, or cook.

According to the FDA, some food companies are making progress; however, the overall amount of sodium in the food supply remains high. One reason is that most of the efforts have focused on making a few foods very low in sodium, rather than making most foods a little lower in sodium.

If the taste keeps you from switching to low-sodium options, there's good news: about two to three months after people start eating less salt, their sense of taste adjusts, and they become more sensitive to low-sodium foods and more satisfied with the flavor.

Figure 7: Paleolithic-era diet vs. modern mineral consumption

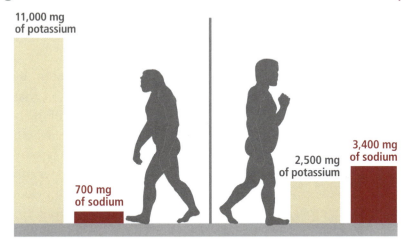

Tens of thousands of years ago, during the Paleolithic period, our ancestors survived on wild animals and a variety of plants—fruits, vegetables, nuts, seeds, roots, leaves, and flowers. The so-called Paleolithic diet delivered plenty of potassium but scant sodium.

Today's typical American diet stands in sharp contrast, packed with processed foods full of white flour, fat, salt, and sugar, as well as meat and dairy products, but with a relative dearth of fruits and vegetables. Some experts blame many of our present-day chronic ailments—including hypertension—on our modern diet, which is at odds with our evolutionary past. Of course, for most people, it's impractical (if not impossible) to eat like a caveman really would have, but you can move toward rebalancing your potassium-sodium ratio with careful food choices (see Table 8, page 39).

SPECIAL SECTION | Conquering your salt habit

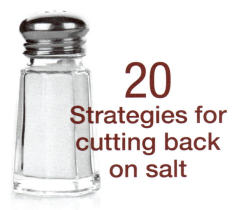

20 Strategies for cutting back on salt

The Department of Nutrition at the Harvard T.H. Chan School of Public Health teamed up with the Culinary Institute of America, a leader in teaching chefs and other food service workers, to create science-based strategies for reducing salt intake. The following list features 20 of those tips, many of which offer a "stealth health" approach to sodium reduction—ways to lower sodium with little or no change to consumer food experiences or choices. Others suggest ways to rebalance and reimagine food choices as well as introduce new foods that can easily translate into satisfying meals. And as a bonus: not only is following these guidelines good for your blood pressure, but it's also an important step to overall health. You can read the full report, *Tasting Success with Cutting Salt*, at www.health.harvard.edu/hsph-cia-sodium.

The big picture: Total diet focus

1 **Downsize your portions.** A good rule of thumb is that the more calories a meal has, the more sodium it has. Two out of three Americans need to lose weight. So skip the supersize. Share a dish when dining out. You can cut your salt—and trim your waist at the same time.

2 **Fill half your plate with fruits and vegetables.** Our bodies need more potassium than sodium. But most Americans' diets provide just the opposite, which can contribute to high blood pressure. Fruits and vegetables are naturally low in sodium—and many fruits and vegetables are good sources of potassium. Filling your plate with them will boost your potassium and shift the sodium-potassium balance in your favor.

3 **Choose foods that are unprocessed or minimally processed.** Processed foods and prepared foods are the greatest sources of sodium in the American diet (75% by some estimates). By choosing fresh foods, you avoid excess sodium being introduced into your diet. Processed, cured meats typically have much more sodium than fresh meats, and canned vegetables usually have more sodium than fresh vegetables. Going easy on processed foods makes sense for general good health, as processing often leads to a loss of nutrients and other benefits of whole or semi-intact foods.

4 **Embrace healthy fats and oils.** Unfortunately, the big low-fat and no-fat product push in the 1990s wasn't rooted in sound science. Many well-meaning product developers cut both the good and bad fats out of formulations, and in order to maintain consumer acceptance of their products, they increased levels of sugar and sodium. So skip most fat-free salad dressings and other similar products, and you'll be doing your blood pressure a favor.

Salt, perception, and psychology

5 **Practice stealth health.** For many foods and preparations, the average person can't detect moderate to substantial differences in sodium levels, including reductions of as much as 25%. Many food manufacturers and restaurant companies have already made or are in the process of making substantial cuts in sodium—some all at once and some over time—that their customers will not be able to detect. Read labels, and opt for lower-sodium versions of the same foods.

6 **Retrain your taste buds.** Studies have found that we can shift our sense of taste to enjoy foods with noticeably lower levels of sodium. One key to success: make the changes gradually and consistently over a period of time, rather than trying to cut back by a large amount all at once (unless of course you find that an immediate 25% reduction in sodium doesn't undermine your enjoyment of a particular food). Try this trick: combine a reduced-sodium version of a favorite product (e.g., vegetable soup) with a regular version in proportions that gradually favor the reduced-sodium version. As time goes on, you won't miss the salt.

Buyer beware: Know your salt facts, ask questions

7 **Target high-volume sodium sources.** Know which ingredients and individual foods are high in sodium, and eat them sparingly. Understand which categories of foods contribute the most sodium to our diets through repeated daily and weekly consumption. Salt is ubiquitous in the American diet, but the top 10 list of food sources of sodium in the U.S. diet is a good place to focus (see "Where's the salt?" on page 36). Choose carefully when buying foods in these categories and eat less of them. Table 9 (page 41) lists more healthful, lower-salt alternatives.

In addition to the prepared foods in the top 10 list, some popular condiments—such as soy sauce, adobo sauce, and certain hot sauces—are very high in sodium. For example, one national brand of soy sauce contains 920 mg of sodium per 1-tablespoon serving, or a whopping 38% of the Daily Value for this nutrient. The "less sodium" version contains 575 mg of sodium, or 24% of the Daily Value.

8 **Scan labels to find foods with less than 150 mg of sodium per serving.** Canned, boxed, frozen, and prepared foods can be high in sodium. Check the label for sodium amounts and choose foods that have less than

Table 8: The power of potassium

Most people eat too much sodium and not enough potassium. To counteract this, eat more foods with a high potassium-to-sodium ratio, like those in the top two-thirds of this chart.

FOOD	POTASSIUM-TO-SODIUM RATIO	CALORIES
Banana (1 medium)	422 to 1	89
Black beans, cooked without salt (½ cup)	305 to 1	109
Orange (1 medium)	232 to 1	69
Grapefruit juice (4 ounces)	126 to 1	48
White beans, cooked without salt (½ cup)	100 to 1	124
Peanuts, dry roasted, no salt (1 ounce)	93 to 1	166
Soybeans, edamame, cooked (½ cup)	72 to 1	95
Avocado (¼ fruit)	69 to 1	57
Raisins (1 small box, 1.5 ounces)	64 to 1	129
Baked potato, plain, with skin (1 medium)	54 to 1	198
Tomato (1 medium)	49 to 1	22
Brussels sprouts, steamed (½ cup)	35 to 1	33
Applesauce, no salt (½ cup)	31 to 1	51
Oatmeal, regular, cooked (⅓ cup)	18 to 1	102
Cantaloupe, cubed (1 cup)	17 to 1	54
Tomato paste, no added salt (¼ cup)	17 to 1	54
Sweet potato, baked (1 medium)	13 to 1	103
Halibut, baked (3 ounces)	8 to 1	94
Spinach, boiled (½ cup)	7 to 1	21
Salmon, baked (3 ounces)	3 to 1	144
Carrots, raw (8 to 10 "baby"-sized)	3 to 1	36
Milk, 1% (1 cup)	3 to 1	102
Yogurt, plain, low-fat (8 ounces)	3 to 1	154
Fast-food French fries, McDonald's (small serving)	2.5 to 1	229
Applesauce, with salt (½ cup)	2.2 to 1	51
Cheerios (1 cup)	1 to 1	106
Salmon, canned (3 ounces)	0.8 to 1	142
Marinara sauce, prepared (½ cup)	0.8 to 1	65
Peanuts, dry roasted, with salt (1 ounce)	0.8 to 1	166
Pork and beans, canned (½ cup)	0.7 to 1	134
Quaker's Instant Oatmeal (1 packet)	0.5 to 1	150
Fast-food cheeseburger	0.4 to 1	280
French bread (1 medium slice)	0.2 to 1	185
Cornflakes (1 cup)	0.2 to 1	100

SPECIAL SECTION | Conquering your salt habit

150 mg per serving (see Table 10, page 42). But pay attention to serving sizes, as they are often unrealistically small. A good rule of thumb for label reading is to look for no more than 1 mg of sodium per calorie of food. You may be surprised to find foods that are high in sodium but that don't list "salt" in the ingredients. That's because there are forms of sodium other than salt (sodium chloride) that are often used in food processing. Examples of these ingredients are monosodium glutamate, sodium citrate, sodium bicarbonate, and sodium alginate.

9 Compare sodium levels on similar grocery items. Compare brands of processed food, including breads, cured meats, cheeses, snack foods, and other foods, choosing those with the lowest levels of sodium that still taste good. Make sure to compare the same serving size. You'll find that there's a surprising degree of variation from brand to brand, since some food manufacturers have made great strides toward cutting the sodium levels in their products. Campbell's, for example, now makes two versions of its V8 drink; the low-sodium version has 75% less sodium than regular V8 juice. Other manufacturers never added much sodium in the first place.

10 Beware of hidden sodium. "Fresh" and "natural" meats and poultry may be injected with salt solutions as part of their processing, and manufacturers are not required to list the sodium content on the label. The best way to find out whether your favorite brand has been treated with a salt solution is to ask the grocer or butcher, or to call the toll-free consumer hotline on the product's label. Some foods that are high in sodium may not taste especially salty, such as breakfast cereals, bakery muffins, energy drinks, and sports drinks.

11 Seek low-sodium menu options when dining out. At the upper end of the spectrum, some chain restaurant and fast-food meals can top 5,000 to 6,000 mg of sodium. It is common to find sandwiches and fast-food entrees with 2,000 to 2,500 mg of sodium each—as much as or more than a day's recommended sodium intake. With food service (or food away from home) now accounting for nearly 50% of the consumer food dollar, both food service and food manufacturing—together with consumers and home cooks—need to be part of the solution to the sodium reduction challenge.

Some tips for consumers: Sodium levels can vary widely from one dish to another and from one restaurant to another. Check restaurant websites for sodium information before you head out, or ask your server to steer you to low-sodium choices. You can also search for your favorite dishes at the Calorie King website (www.calorieking.com), which includes nutrient data for foods from hundreds of popular nationwide chains. Federal law now requires all restaurants with more than 20 locations to provide this information. Increasingly, chain restaurants are responding to calls for sodium reduction, so watch for news about such initiatives by your favorite restaurant group.

Certain cuisines tend to have higher sodium levels than others. Asian restaurants use a lot of sodium-rich soy and fish sauces, and Italian food (especially pizza) features high-sodium sauces, cheeses, and cured meats, such as pepperoni and prosciutto. A better option (if available) is a "farm-to-table" restaurant. These fashionable eateries focus on fresh and often locally grown or raised foods. While they may not provide nutritional information, these establishments—as well as other neighborhood and smaller "mom-and-pop" places—may be willing to work with you to prepare a lower-sodium meal. These days, with more people following gluten-free and vegan diets, they're often used to making adjustments. And it's in their best interest to make their customers happy.

If you're comfortable doing so, tell your server you have a medical condition or are taking medication and need to limit your salt. He or she may be more inclined to take you seriously. Then say, "Please tell the chef to grill, broil, or steam my food with no added seasonings or sauces."

If you've got your heart set on an entree that's over your sodium budget, ask the server to box up half of the dish to save for the next day before bringing it to your table. That way, you can enjoy the portion without being tempted to pick at the rest just because it's in front of you. Save high-salt choices for very limited special occasions.

Flavor strategies and culinary insights

12 Consider flavor as a new health imperative. The national conversation about salt and sodium should not be just about salty taste and sodium reduction, but about flavor in general. For too long, the national food and agricultural focus has been on quantity and value—and quality often as a function of consistency, appearance, safety, convenience, and shelf life. If natural flavor sometimes suffered, there was always fat, sugar, and salt to take up the slack—all high-impact, low-cost flavor enhancers that most people love. But at a time when we have "over-delivered" on the promise of affordable calories, and both salt and sugar (and all refined carbohydrates) have turned out to have harmful health consequences, we need to refocus our attention on enhancing natural flavors.

13 Know your seasons, and, even better, your local farmer. Shop for raw ingredients

Table 9: Lower-sodium alternatives

Sodium levels can vary widely within similar food categories, and even foods that don't seem salty, such as milk shakes and licorice, may be high in sodium. This table can help you choose lower-sodium options among common food categories. (Note that the serving sizes represent quantities people typically eat and are not always the same between low- and high-sodium choices.)

FOOD CATEGORY	LOW	SODIUM (MG)	HIGH	SODIUM (MG)
Dairy products	Milk, 2% fat (1 cup)	127	Cottage cheese, 2% fat (1 cup)	746
	Swiss cheese (1 ounce)	10	Parmesan cheese, hard (1 ounce)	390
	Breyers Natural Vanilla ice cream (½ cup)	17	McDonald's Chocolate McCafé Shake (small, 12 fluid ounces)	260
Fruits and vegetables	Asparagus, fresh steamed (½ cup)	13	Asparagus, canned (½ cup)	347
	Orange juice (1 cup)	2	V8 100% Vegetable Juice (1 cup)	640
	Contadina Tomato Sauce, No Salt Added (½ cup)	20	Contadina Tomato Sauce, regular (½ cup)	560
Meat and fish	Halibut (3 ounces)	58	Alaskan king crab (3 ounces)	911
	Chicken, broiler or fryer, white meat (3 ounces)	55	Oscar Mayer Deli Fresh Oven Roasted Turkey Breast (2 ounces)	540
	Ground beef, 90% lean (3 ounces)	56	Hebrew National Beef Franks (1 link)	450
Cereals and grains	Kashi Cinnamon Harvest cereal (28 biscuits)	0	Kellogg's Raisin Bran (1 cup)	210
	Post Spoon Size Shredded Wheat (1 cup)	0	General Mills Cheerios (1 cup)	140
	Flahavan's Irish Steel Cut Oatmeal, cooked, no salt added (⅓ cup)	0	Oat bran muffin (1 medium)	444
Candy, snacks, condiments	Gummi Bear candies (17 pieces)	10	Twizzlers black licorice (4 strands)	200
	Silver Palate Salad Splash dressing, Balsamic Country (2 tablespoons)	15	Wish-Bone Italian salad dressing (2 tablespoons)	340
	Garden of Eatin' Blue Chips, No Salt Added, blue corn tortilla chips (1 ounce)	10	Utz Sourdough Specials, pretzels, extra dark (1 ounce)	470

SPECIAL SECTION | Conquering your salt habit

Table 10: Reading food labels

To assess a food's sodium level, check the back and sides as well as the front of the package or container. The label on the front may offer a clue (see below for a translation of what the terms mean). But the actual amount is listed in the Nutrition Facts panel (at right), found on the product's back or side.

IF THE LABEL SAYS:	IT MEANS:
Sodium-free or salt-free	Less than 5 mg sodium per serving
Very low sodium	Less than 35 mg sodium per serving
Low sodium	Less than 140 mg sodium per serving
Reduced sodium	At least 25% less sodium than original product
Light in sodium	At least 50% less sodium than original product
Unsalted or no added salt	No salt added during processing (not necessarily sodium-free)

with maximum natural flavor, thereby avoiding the need to add as much (if any) sodium. Seek out peak-of-season produce from farmers' markets and your local supermarket.

14 Spice it up. One of the easiest ways to reduce the need for added salt is through the use of ingredients such as spices, dried and fresh herbs, roots (such as garlic and ginger), citrus, vinegars, and wine. From black pepper, cinnamon, and turmeric to fresh basil, chili peppers, and lemon juice, these flavor enhancers create excitement on the palate—and can do it with less sodium. Use cayenne, paprika, parsley, sage, rosemary, or thyme for meats; caraway, basil, dill, marjoram, nutmeg, parsley, sage, or thyme with vegetables; cinnamon, cloves, ginger, or nutmeg with fruit. The possibilities are endless. (For more ideas, see "Salt swaps" on page 43.) In addition to introducing you to new tastes, using more herbs and spices will give you extra phytonutrients that have been linked to reductions in risk of cancer, diabetes, and other chronic conditions.

15 Go nuts for healthy fats in the kitchen. As chefs and home cooks know, fat is a great carrier and enhancer of flavor. Using the right healthy fats—from roasted nuts and avocados to vegetable oils, such as olive, canola, or soybean oil—can help make up for any flavor loss from using less salt. Some healthy fats contribute their own flavors (think peanut butter and extra-virgin olive oil), while other fats help to juice up flavor in pan searing and frying.

16 Use umami to boost flavor. Umami (pronounced oo-MAH-me), or savoriness, is the so-called "fifth taste" that in recent years sensory scientists have brought into the mainstream of academic research. Foods that are naturally high in a compound called L-glutamate trigger our umami taste receptors. Cooked chicken, fish, beef, and soybeans are naturally high in umami, as are mushrooms, tomatoes, seaweed, carrots, and Chinese cabbage. Incorporating these foods into meals can add a delicious depth of flavor without adding salt.

17 Sear, sauté, and roast to help spare the salt. Take the time to learn some simple techniques that can make your cooking less reliant on sodium. Searing and sautéing foods in a pan builds flavor (try searing umami-rich mushrooms in a hot pan with oil). Roasting brings out the natural sweetness of many vegetables and the savoriness of fish and chicken. Steaming and microwaving tend to dilute flavors; perk up steamed dishes with a finishing drizzle of flavorful oil and a squeeze of citrus.

18 Be careful how you use your daily sodium allowance. Consider your sodium budget—1,500 mg per day if you have high blood pressure, and 2,300 mg daily if you don't. Then decide which foods to "spend" it on. You will have greater success if you use it to enhance the flavors of vegetables, whole grains, nuts, legumes, and other healthy ingredients versus "overspending" it on salty snacks, heavily processed food, high-sodium fast foods, and other foods that we should be consuming in smaller amounts. Rethink that double bacon cheeseburger or the breakfast special with ham and sausage.

19 Discover a world of ideas for flavor development. Look to global culinary traditions—from Europe and the Mediterranean, Latin America, Asia, and Africa—for ways to transform fruits, vegetables, and other healthy ingredients into exciting flavors and meals. Because many of these world culinary traditions build up flavor in novel, complex, and intriguing ways, cooks are under less pressure to use as much sodium. Sometimes these flavors will appear in higher-sodium versions, but the culinary ideas for lower-sodium strategies are still there, embedded in traditional cultural approaches to flavor development that go way beyond fat, salt, and sugar (our all-too-frequent default flavor enhancers in the United States).

20 Go beyond bread and sandwiches for whole grains. Collectively, because we eat so much of it, bread is one of the largest contributors of sodium to our diets. Even whole-grain bread, while a healthier choice than white, can contain considerable sodium. But only part of the sodium in bread is for taste: much of it is used to help the bread-making process and preserve the final results. You can skip that extra sodium when you use whole grains—such as quinoa or brown rice—by themselves.

Salt swaps

Because salt-laden restaurant fare and processed foods are by far the biggest sources of salt in our diets, eating home-cooked foods is the most effective strategy for cutting back. In the kitchen, swapping regular salt for sodium-free or lower-sodium alternatives can help. Here are some options.

Lemon, lime, vinegar

Instead of salt, try fresh lemon juice, lime juice, or flavored vinegars to brighten taste.

Herb and spice blends

Many people like salt-free herb and spice blends, which come in more than a dozen different flavors. Popular brands include Mrs. Dash, Penzeys salt-free spice blends, or salt-free Spike. You can also make your own blend by mixing the following:

- 1 teaspoon each of dried basil, oregano, marjoram, thyme, and dill
- ¼ teaspoon each of savory, sage, onion powder, and garlic powder
- ⅛ teaspoon of powdered ginger.

No-sodium salts

Potassium-based salt substitutes, such as AlsoSalt, Morton Salt Substitute, NoSalt, and Nu-Salt, are a good option for many people, especially since increasing your potassium intake can help lower blood pressure. But people who have kidney damage or who take drugs that increase potassium levels should avoid them (see "A warning on potassium pills and salt substitutes," page 31).

Low-sodium salts

Products that combine salt and potassium chloride, such as Morton Lite Salt, are another option. Note that sea salt and kosher salt are not low-sodium alternatives; they have about the same amount of sodium as regular table salt.

Lighter flakes

You can also find reduced-sodium salt that's made into flake-shaped crystals, which are less dense and therefore lower in sodium by volume (Diamond Crystal Salt Sense).

For example, try a Mediterranean-inspired whole-grain salad with chopped vegetables, nuts, and legumes, perhaps a small amount of cheese, herbs and spices, and healthy oils and vinegar or citrus. For breakfast, cook steel-cut oats, farro, or other intact whole grains with a generous amount of fresh or dried fruit, and you can skip the toast (and the extra sodium). ♥

Medications for lowering blood pressure

Doctors once hesitated to prescribe medication until a person's blood pressure reached 160/100 mm Hg. Anything below that level was deemed "mild hypertension" and was not considered dangerous. As a result, many doctors worried that the drugs' potential side effects might outweigh their benefits. These perceptions turned out to be false. Research clearly shows the value of using drugs, if necessary, to treat blood pressure once it reaches Stage 1 hypertension (130/80 to 139/90 mm Hg) or higher.

Today, blood pressure can be controlled with lower doses of medications, meaning there is less chance of side effects. Doctors can choose from among more than 200 drugs—called antihypertensive medications—to treat high blood pressure, including many preparations that combine two or more drugs. Many newer antihypertensive drugs have a slightly different chemical structure from older drugs but produce nearly identical effects in the body. Others act in entirely different ways. Doctors can tailor treatment to the individual person and can often prescribe a drug that controls blood pressure, produces few or no side effects, and, hopefully, protects against complications. In addition, it's often possible to use a single medication to treat both high blood pressure and accompanying medical problems, like heart failure.

Among this vast array, no single drug is inherently superior to the others. Blood pressure control is ultimately a numbers game: the value of any blood pressure drug is judged on an individual basis, depending on how much the medication reduces blood pressure for the person who takes it and how well it protects against damage to the heart, brain, kidneys, and eyes caused by high blood pressure.

Experts recommend starting any drug to lower blood pressure at the lowest possible dose and gradually increasing it until blood pressure sinks to a normal level. If the drug causes troublesome side effects, the dosage should be reduced, or it should be replaced with a different medication.

The usual course of treatment for Stage 1 hypertension is to begin with one drug and add a second if your blood pressure does not fall to desired levels. You may have to try several medications before you find a drug, or a combination, that works. The treatment for Stage 2 hypertension often begins with a two-drug combination. You may need more than one or two drugs if your blood pressure doesn't drop to an acceptable level. With all stages of hypertension, lifestyle changes are always an important component of treatment.

Table 11: ACE inhibitors

GENERIC NAME	BRAND NAME	SIDE EFFECTS
benazepril	Lotensin	Cough, rash, fluid retention, high potassium levels, and loss of taste. Possible low blood pressure and fainting. Swelling of the lips, tongue, and throat (angioedema). Can worsen kidney function if narrowed arteries feed both kidneys. May cause miscarriage; should never be used during pregnancy or in women intending to become pregnant.
captopril	Capoten	
enalapril	Vasotec	
fosinopril	Monopril	
lisinopril	Prinivil, Zestril	
quinapril	Accupril	
ramipril	Altace	

Table 12: Angiotensin-receptor blockers (ARBs)

GENERIC NAME	BRAND NAME	SIDE EFFECTS
azilsartan medoxomil	Edarbi	Muscle cramps, dizziness. Swelling of the lips, tongue, and throat (angioedema). Should never be used during pregnancy or in women intending to become pregnant.
candesartan	Atacand	
eprosartan	Teveten	
irbesartan	Avapro	
losartan	Cozaar	
olmesartan	Benicar	
telmisartan	Micardis	
valsartan	Diovan	

Classes of drugs to lower blood pressure

Several classes of drugs are available to fight high blood pressure: angiotensin-converting–enzyme (ACE) inhibitors, angiotensin-receptor blockers (ARBs), direct renin inhibitors, diuretics, calcium-channel blockers, anti-adrenergics, and direct-acting vasodilators. In addition, researchers are testing two other potent classes: aldosterone synthetase inhibitors and vasopeptidase inhibitors. With so many choices available, which medication should you and your doctor choose? The 2017 blood pressure guidelines say that for people with Stage 1 high blood pressure, first-line therapy can include drugs from these common four classes: thiazide diuretics, calcium-channel blockers, ACE inhibitors, and ARBs.

For people with Stage 2 high blood pressure, the guidelines recommend starting with two first-line drugs of different classes. The best drug or combination of drugs for you will depend on your risk of heart disease and any other medical conditions you may have (see "The right drug for the right person," page 50).

ACE inhibitors

Drugs in this class prevent the kidneys from retaining sodium and water by deactivating angiotensin-converting enzyme (ACE), which converts inactive angiotensin I to the active angiotensin II (see Figure 2, page 5). Angiotensin II raises blood pressure by triggering sodium and water retention and constricting the arteries.

ACE inhibitors (see Table 11, page 44) reduce blood pressure in most people and produce fewer side effects than many other antihypertensive drugs. In addition, ACE inhibitors protect the kidneys of people with diabetes and kidney dysfunction and the hearts of people with heart failure.

The most common side effects of these drugs are a reduced sense of taste and a dry cough. Occasionally, people taking ACE inhibitors develop angioedema, which causes the lips, tongue, and throat to swell. Although this side effect is not that common, it can trigger serious breathing problems, so tell your doctor immediately if you notice it. ACE inhibitors can also cause potassium retention, so people with poor kidney function must use them cautiously. Because these drugs can cause miscarriage, women who are pregnant or trying to get pregnant should not take them.

Table 13: Diuretics

CLASS	GENERIC NAME	BRAND NAME	SIDE EFFECTS
Thiazide diuretics	chlorothiazide	Diuril	Weakness, confusion, potassium depletion, gout, fatigue, thirst, frequent urination, lightheadedness, muscle cramps, diarrhea or constipation, increased sensitivity to sunlight, allergic reaction in people allergic to sulfa drugs, impotence, high blood sugar, elevated cholesterol.
	chlorthalidone	Hygroton	
	hydrochlorothiazide	Esidrix, HydroDiuril, Microzide	
	indapamide	Lozol	
	metolazone	Diulo, Mykrox, Zaroxolyn	
Loop diuretics	bumetanide	Bumex	Weakness, confusion, potassium depletion, gout, fatigue, thirst, diarrhea or constipation, increased sensitivity to sunlight, allergic reaction in people allergic to sulfa drugs, impotence.
	ethacrynic acid	Edecrin	
	furosemide	Lasix	
	torsemide	Demadex	
Potassium-sparing diuretics/aldosterone-receptor blockers*	amiloride	Midamor	Excessive potassium levels, especially in people with kidney disease; breast enlargement and erectile dysfunction in men; menstrual irregularities and breast enlargement or tenderness in women, headache, dizziness, diarrhea, fatigue, upset stomach.
	eplerenone	Inspra	
	spironolactone	Aldactone	
	triamterene	Dyrenium	

*Note: Potassium-sparing diuretics directly or indirectly block aldosterone, a hormone that raises blood pressure by causing the kidneys to conserve sodium and water. As a result, these four medications are sometimes also known as aldosterone-receptor blockers. They also affect other hormones and thus carry some unwanted side effects, such as breast enlargement and impotence in men and menstrual irregularities in women.

Table 14: Calcium-channel blockers

GENERIC NAME	BRAND NAME	SIDE EFFECTS
amlodipine	Norvasc	Headache, dizziness, edema, and heartburn. Nifedipine can cause palpitations. Diltiazem and verapamil can cause constipation and a slowed heartbeat.
diltiazem	Cardizem, Dilacor, others	
felodipine	Plendil	
isradipine	DynaCirc	
nicardipine	Cardene, Cardene SR	
nifedipine	Adalat CC, Procardia XL	
verapamil	Calan, Isoptin, others	

Angiotensin-receptor blockers (ARBs)

Like ACE inhibitors, angiotensin-receptor blockers lower blood pressure by relaxing blood vessels and preventing the kidneys from retaining sodium and water—but rather than preventing the formation of angiotensin II in the first place, they hinder its action by blocking receptors for it in the blood vessels. Because ARBs are highly effective and well tolerated by most people who take them, these medications have become quite popular (see Table 12, page 44). They don't produce any of the traditional side effects of other antihypertensive medications, and they're less likely than ACE inhibitors to cause a cough. In addition, like ACE inhibitors, they benefit people with diabetes, heart failure, or both.

Direct renin inhibitors

These drugs work by inhibiting the activity of renin, the enzyme largely responsible for angiotensin II levels. In clinical trials, renin inhibitors have proven effective in not only lowering blood pressure, but also keeping blood pressure levels steadier throughout the day. (Fluctuations throughout the day have been linked with heart problems.) One renin inhibitor, aliskiren (Tekturna), has been approved by the FDA. Like ACE inhibitors and ARBs, it should never be used during pregnancy.

Diuretics

Diuretics, commonly called "water pills," are the oldest and least expensive class of drugs used to treat hypertension (see Table 13, page 45). They help the kidneys eliminate sodium and water from the body. This process decreases blood volume, which in turn lowers blood pressure. There are several types of diuretics:

- Loop diuretics, which act on the part of the kidney tubules called the loop of Henle, block sodium and chloride from being reabsorbed from the tubules into the bloodstream.
- Thiazide diuretics act on another portion of the kidney tubules to stop sodium from re-entering circulation.
- Potassium-sparing diuretics help counteract one drawback of other diuretics, which is that they deplete potassium, so that people taking them frequently need to take potassium supplements as well. Potassium-sparing diuretics solve that problem, but by the same token, they can cause dangerously high levels of potassium in some people.

Diuretics are especially effective for salt-sensitive people with high blood pressure and older people with isolated systolic hypertension. Aside from treating hypertension, diuretics are often prescribed for fluid retention (edema) caused by heart failure,

▶ Tips for taking diuretics

Needing to urinate more frequently when you take diuretics can interfere with sleep and outings. It can also lead to dehydration if you don't pay attention to keeping your fluid level in balance. Although these side effects can be inconvenient, don't be tempted to skip pills or stop taking them. Here are some tips to help you manage your medicines.

- Pay attention to how soon you need to urinate after taking your pill. Plan your trips away from home for when your medicine is less active.
- Find out where the bathroom is when you go to a new place. This will save time and hassles when you have to go.
- Don't skip your medicine when you're on vacation.
- Since your diuretic will be most active in the first two or three hours, take your pill in the morning to avoid having to wake up to use the bathroom during the night.
- If you take two doses, take your second pill by 4 p.m. This allows several hours for the diuretic to work before bedtime.
- Tell your doctor if you notice any signs of dehydration such as dizziness, extreme thirst, dark urine, low urine output, very dry mouth, or constipation.

kidney disorders, liver disease, or premenstrual bloating.

Perhaps the most common side effect of diuretics is frequent urination, which can be particularly bothersome (see "Tips for taking diuretics," page 46, for advice on coping with this problem). Other side effects include lightheadedness, fatigue, diarrhea or constipation, and muscle cramps. Men may occasionally experience erectile dysfunction. Diuretics can cause gout, a painful form of arthritis caused by the buildup of uric acid in the body, because they elevate blood levels of this substance.

In addition, thiazide diuretics can raise blood sugar levels. In some people, this may be enough to cause diabetes or make their diabetes worse. That's why blood sugar should be monitored in people taking a diuretic for blood pressure control.

Calcium-channel blockers

Calcium-channel blockers (see Table 14, page 46) slow the movement of calcium into the smooth-muscle cells of the heart and blood vessels. This alters heart muscle contractions and dilates blood vessels, lowering blood pressure. Because calcium-channel blockers also slow nerve impulses in the heart, they are often prescribed for irregular heartbeat (arrhythmias). Common side effects of calcium-channel blockers are headaches, swelling, heartburn, slow heart rate (bradycardia), and constipation.

Anti-adrenergics

Anti-adrenergics lower blood pressure by limiting the action of the neurotransmitters epinephrine and norepinephrine, thereby relaxing the blood vessels and reducing the speed and force of the heart's contractions. (Epinephrine and norepinephrine are sometimes called adrenaline and noradrenaline—hence the name anti-adrenergics.) This class includes a variety of different agents that work in slightly different ways (see Table 15, above).

Table 15: Anti-adrenergic drugs

CLASS	GENERIC NAME	BRAND NAME	SIDE EFFECTS
Beta blockers (cardio-selective)	acebutolol	Sectral	Wheezing, dizziness, depression, impotence, fatigue, insomnia, decreased HDL cholesterol levels, lower exercise tolerance. Can worsen peripheral vascular disease and heart failure. Abrupt withdrawal may trigger angina or a heart attack in people with heart disease.
	atenolol	Tenormin	
	betaxolol	Kerlone	
	bisoprolol	Zebeta	
	metoprolol	Lopressor, Toprol-XL	
	nebivolol	Bystolic	
	penbutolol	Levatol	
Beta blockers (non-selective)	nadolol	Corgard	
	pindolol	Visken	
	propranolol	Inderal, Inderal LA	
	sotalol	Betapace, Sorine	
	timolol	Blocadren	
Alpha-1 blockers	doxazosin	Cardura	A drop in blood pressure upon standing up, fainting, weakness, heart palpitations, headache, nasal congestion, dry mouth.
	prazosin	Minipress	
	terazosin	Hytrin	
Alpha and beta blockers	carvedilol	Coreg	Wheezing, depression, insomnia, diarrhea, lightheadedness, dizziness, unusual tiredness or weakness, drying of the eyes, erectile dysfunction, headache, dry mouth, nasal congestion, decreased HDL cholesterol levels, lower exercise tolerance, a drop in blood pressure upon standing up, fainting, heart palpitations. Can worsen peripheral vascular disease and heart failure. Abrupt withdrawal may trigger angina or a heart attack in people with heart disease.
	labetalol	Normodyne, Trandate	
Centrally acting agents	clonidine	Catapres, Catapres-TTS	A drop in blood pressure upon standing up, drowsiness, sedation, dry mouth, fatigue, erectile dysfunction, depression, dizziness. Catapres-TTS (a patch) may cause a rash.
	methyldopa	Aldomet	
Peripheral nerve-acting agents	guanethidine	Ismelin	A drop in blood pressure upon standing up, depression, nasal stuffiness, nightmares. Guanethidine may slow heart rate, and reserpine may cause indigestion.
	reserpine	Serpalan	

> ### Receptor blockers: Fooling the body
>
> The discovery of the "lock and key" system of cell communication opened the door to a new world of drug research. The search began with a simple question: why do some cells react to particular chemicals, but not others? The answer is both maddeningly complex and extremely simple.
>
> Chemicals circulating through the blood, such as hormones and neurotransmitters, stimulate cells. At any given moment, a cell may come in contact with hundreds of different chemicals, so it must be selective about which ones it responds to. To do this, cells have special structures on their outer surfaces called receptors. A receptor operates much like a car's ignition switch. Only a chemical with the right molecular configuration (the key) will fit the receptor (the lock) and start up biological activity inside the cell.
>
> Researchers have used their knowledge of this system to formulate drugs that prevent cells from responding to certain substances. Beta blockers, which are used to treat high blood pressure, are a prime example. At times of stress and during exercise, your nerve cells release the neurotransmitters epinephrine and norepinephrine. When epinephrine attaches to beta receptors on cells in your heart, the heart cells become activated, increasing your heart rate and the strength of your heart's contractions. This raises your blood pressure. But beta blockers attach to the same receptors, because their structure has been carefully designed to fit neatly into the same "lock." With this spot filled, epinephrine and norepinephrine can't connect to the receptor, thus breaking the chain of chemical communication that would otherwise stimulate the heart and spark an increase in blood pressure.

Peripheral adrenergic-receptor blockers. These drugs work by preventing neurotransmitters from attaching to cells and stimulating the heart and blood vessels. They are divided into two major groups: beta blockers and alpha blockers.

Beta blockers, which have been used since the 1960s, lock on to cell structures called beta receptors—the same receptors that certain neurotransmitters (primarily epinephrine) normally attach themselves to in order to stimulate the heart (see "Receptor blockers: Fooling the body," above). Thus, by preventing the neurotransmitters from activating heart cells, beta blockers cause the heart rate to slow and blood pressure to fall. More than a dozen beta blockers have been approved for use in the United States (see Table 15, page 47). They fall into three main groups—nonselective, cardioselective, and third-generation.

- Nonselective beta blockers, like propranolol (Inderal), were the earliest. These affect both beta-1 receptors, found in heart cells, and beta-2 receptors, found in the lungs and blood vessels. They should be used with caution, if at all, in smokers or people with asthma or other lung conditions.
- Cardioselective beta blockers, including atenolol (Tenormin) and metoprolol (Toprol, Lopressor), were designed to block only beta-1 receptors. Since they don't affect beta-2 receptors, cardioselective beta blockers are safer for people with lung disorders.
- Third-generation beta blockers do more than block beta receptors. Labetalol (Normodyne, Trandate) and carvedilol (Coreg) block alpha receptors, too. This further helps relax blood vessels. Nebivolol (Bystolic) stimulates the inner lining of blood vessels (the endothelium) to generate nitric oxide, which helps the vessels relax.

All beta blockers can worsen asthma or other chronic lung disorders, but the nonselective agents are potentially more dangerous for people with respiratory problems. Beta blockers can also worsen heart failure in some people while improving it in others. They can mask the warning signs of hypoglycemia (low blood sugar) in people with diabetes. The most common side effects of beta blockers are fatigue, depression, erectile dysfunction, shortness of breath, insomnia, and reduced tolerance for exercise.

Alpha blockers are similar in action to beta blockers, but they work on alpha-1 receptors in the heart and blood vessels—the sites where neurotransmitters that cause vessel constriction (primarily norepinephrine) attach themselves. In addition to

Table 16: Direct-acting vasodilators

GENERIC NAME	BRAND NAME	SIDE EFFECTS
hydralazine	Apresoline	Headaches, palpitations, weakness, flushing, nausea. Minoxidil may cause hair growth, fluid retention, and increased blood sugar.
minoxidil	Loniten	

reducing blood pressure, alpha-1 blockers also reduce "bad" LDL cholesterol levels and increase "good" HDL cholesterol, making these drugs especially useful for hypertensive people with cholesterol problems. They may also improve insulin sensitivity in people with glucose intolerance and hyperglycemia (high blood sugar). And they are often prescribed for men with benign prostatic hyperplasia, a noncancerous enlargement of the prostate gland, because these drugs relax smooth muscles surrounding the prostate, relieving the constriction of the urethra and easing urine flow.

Side effects of alpha blockers include orthostatic hypotension (a drop in blood pressure upon standing up; see "When blood pressure suddenly drops," page 6), heart palpitations, dizziness, nasal congestion, headaches, and dry mouth. These drugs can also cause erectile dysfunction, although not as frequently as some other blood pressure medications.

Some people require both alpha and beta blockers to control their blood pressure. The drugs labetalol and carvedilol have properties of both.

Centrally acting agents. These agents work by preventing your brain from sending signals to your nervous system to speed up your heart rate and narrow your blood vessels—two activities that boost blood pressure. These drugs include clonidine (Catapres) and methyldopa (Aldomet). Like peripheral nerve–acting agents (see next entry), they are generally used in combination with other blood pressure medicines. Common side effects include abnormally low blood pressure when standing up, dry mouth, depression, erectile dysfunction, and sedation.

Peripheral nerve–acting agents. These antiadrenergics (now used far less often because of frequent side effects) deplete the autonomic nerves of norepinephrine, a substance that causes vessels to contract and raises blood pressure. Such drugs are usually prescribed along with other blood pressure medicines since they are more effective this way. Reserpine (Serpalan) can cause depression, nightmares, nasal stuffiness, and indigestion, while guanethidine (Ismelin) is more apt to bring on orthostatic hypotension and slow the heart rate.

Direct-acting vasodilators

Direct-acting vasodilators (see Table 16, page 48) relax the arteries. They act quickly and are often used in emergencies. However, they can cause fluid retention and tachycardia (fast heart rate), so doctors usually prescribe them in combination with another blood pressure medication that slows the heart rate, such as a cardioselective beta blocker. Hydralazine (Apresoline) and minoxidil (Loniten), the direct-acting vasodila-

> ### Renal denervation for resistant hypertension?
>
> An experimental procedure to treat hypertension is called renal denervation. It involves threading a slender tube (catheter) into the arteries that supply the kidneys. A tiny device at the catheter's tip delivers bursts of energy or sound waves that damage some of the nerves supplying the kidneys, which are involved in blood pressure regulation.
>
> Early studies suggested that renal denervation appeared to be a safe, effective, and lasting way to control high blood pressure. However, the procedure suffered a serious setback in 2014. In a carefully controlled trial, whose 535 participants were taking at least three drugs to control their blood pressure, renal denervation proved no more effective than a sham procedure.
>
> However, subsequent studies suggest that the technique may be effective, and many different designs of special catheters are being tested. But the ultimate usefulness of renal denervation remains unclear for now.

Tips to help you remember to take your blood pressure medicine

- Take your medicine after you brush your teeth. Keep it with your toothpaste as a reminder.
- Put self-stick notes in visible places to remind yourself.
- Use a weekly pillbox to store your medicines so you can see at a glance whether you've taken the current day's dose.
- Keep your medicine on the nightstand next to your bed to remind yourself to take your evening medications.
- Call your voicemail and leave a reminder to take your medicine; then don't erase the message.
- Set a reminder alarm on your cellphone.
- Establish a buddy system with a friend who also takes a medication each day.

tors most commonly used to treat high blood pressure, can cause headaches, weakness, flushing, and nausea. In addition, minoxidil can cause hair growth, fluid retention, and increased blood sugar. (The hair growth side effect of minoxidil was turned into a plus—in a formulation called Rogaine, minoxidil is an FDA-approved drug that slows or stops hair loss and promotes hair regrowth.)

Drug combinations

Because having to take several different pills often presents an obstacle for people sticking to their blood pressure treatment program, some of the most common drug combinations are available in a single pill. Frequently prescribed combination medications include pills in which the diuretic hydrochlorothiazide (often abbreviated as HCT) is added to an ARB such as irbesartan or valsartan or an ACE inhibitor such as benazepril or lisinopril. There are also combinations of ARBs plus the diuretic chlorthalidone. For people who need three drugs to control their blood pressure, there are two drugs that combine an ARB, a calcium-channel blocker, and a diuretic (Exforge HCT and Tribenzor).

The right drug for the right person

If you can't control your blood pressure by adopting healthier habits—such as limiting salt, increasing exercise, and quitting smoking—then it's time for medications. With so many choices available, which one is right for you? That depends on how your body metabolizes medications, any other health conditions you might have, and your pill-taking preferences.

Designing an effective medication program for high blood pressure is like fitting together the pieces of a jigsaw puzzle. Matching the benefits and side effects of the dozens of available drugs to an individual's risk factors, health conditions, and lifestyle considerations is often a trial-and-error process. What may work well for your neighbor or cousin may not be right for you. So talk with your doctor about which medications offer you the best blood pressure control with the fewest side effects. The best regimen should be tailored to your needs and medical history, your preferences about how and when to take medications, and your concerns about side effects. If you have other medical conditions, that also may affect the choice of blood pressure drugs (see Table 17, page 51). Some special considerations apply to African Americans and

Can stress reduction lower your need for medication?

Controlling your stress can help lower your blood pressure. But can it reduce your need to take blood pressure medicine?

To answer this question, investigators conducted a randomized trial to determine the impact of the relaxation response on both blood pressure and the need for medication. (The relaxation response is a physiological state that can be elicited through a variety of mental and physical techniques aimed at reducing stress.) The study involved 122 people ages 55 and over, with systolic blood pressure between 140 and 159 mm Hg, who took at least two blood pressure medications. Participants were divided into two groups: one practiced the relaxation response for eight weeks, and the other received health education about blood pressure.

After eight weeks, 34 of the people who practiced the relaxation response—a little more than half—had lowered their systolic blood pressure by more than 5 mm Hg, and were eligible for the next phase of the study, in which they could reduce levels of the medication they were taking. During that second phase, 50% were able to eliminate at least one blood pressure medicine, and 35% were able to reduce the dosage of their medication.

People in the health education group also saw improvement, although it was not as dramatic as in the relaxation response group. In the education group, 24 people (a little more than a third of those who started) were able to reduce their blood pressure enough to progress to the second phase of the study. During that second phase, 19% eliminated medication, and 50% reduced their dosage.

The study thus demonstrated that both practicing the relaxation response and undergoing health education can let some people reduce systolic pressure by about 10 mm Hg, but those who practiced the relaxation response were more likely to successfully eliminate or reduce their antihypertensive medications. Subsequent studies are planned to examine whether people at risk of developing high blood pressure can use relaxation techniques to stave off full-blown hypertension and the use of medications altogether. While the results of this study are compelling, just remember that any reduction or elimination of medication must be done on your doctor's recommendation and under his or her supervision.

Table 17: Drug advice for people with concurrent health problems

Below are some general guidelines regarding medication choices for people who have other illnesses in addition to high blood pressure.

CONDITION	MEDICATION ADVICE
Coronary artery disease	Beta blockers and calcium-channel blockers often benefit people who have chest pain (angina). For people who've had a heart attack, beta blockers also lower the risk of having another one.
Heart failure	ACE inhibitors help prevent the progression of heart failure. Diuretics, beta blockers, and ARBs may also be beneficial.
Left ventricular hypertrophy (thickening of the heart's left wall)	ACE inhibitors are considered most effective; however, all antihypertensive drugs except direct-acting vasodilators (hydralazine and minoxidil) reduce left ventricle wall thickness.
Kidney disease	ACE inhibitors or ARBs slow the progression of kidney disease. But they can promote a dangerous buildup of potassium, especially when taken with NSAIDs such as ibuprofen and many prescription painkillers. Consequently, potassium levels and kidney function tests must be closely monitored. Loop diuretics help control the fluid buildup common in people with kidney disease; however, potassium-sparing diuretics can be dangerous.
Diabetes	ACE inhibitors or ARBs slow the progression of kidney disease, a possible complication of diabetes. But other antihypertensive drugs can worsen diabetes symptoms. Thiazide diuretics, which may raise blood sugar levels, and beta blockers, which can mask the symptoms of low blood sugar (hypoglycemia), should be used with caution.
High cholesterol	Alpha-1 blockers may slightly reduce total cholesterol and raise levels of protective HDL. But other medications have harmful effects; for example, beta blockers can increase triglyceride levels and reduce beneficial HDL, and high doses of thiazide and loop diuretics can raise overall cholesterol levels, "bad" LDL cholesterol, and triglycerides. Calcium-channel blockers, ACE inhibitors, and ARBs do not affect blood lipids.
Respiratory diseases (asthma, bronchitis, emphysema)	Beta blockers can aggravate the symptoms of respiratory ailments, but most other antihypertensive agents can be used safely. Note that many over-the-counter asthma preparations and cold remedies contain vasoconstrictors, which can raise both heart rate and blood pressure. Consult your doctor before taking these medications.
Gout	Diuretics can increase uric acid levels, making gout attacks more likely. Use these drugs with caution if you have gout.

older people. However, people vary enough in their responses that race or age should not be the principal factor influencing drug selection.

African Americans

Developing healthy habits is particularly important if you are African American, since African Americans in general tend to have higher rates of smoking, obesity, diabetes, and salt sensitivity, plus lower amounts of potassium in the diet. You are also more likely to incur complications such as stroke or kidney damage as a result of unchecked hypertension. Diuretics may work especially well for you because of their effectiveness in treating hypertension in people who are salt-sensitive. Calcium-channel blockers may also be a good choice. By contrast, ACE inhibitors seem to be less effective at low doses when prescribed as a single medication. Ultimately, many African Americans have such severe hypertension that two or more drugs are needed to bring blood pressure under control. But again, individuals can vary widely, so there are no ironclad rules.

Older people or those in poor health

Because many older people have multiple health concerns, their medication regimen should be carefully tailored to account for conditions in addition to hypertension (see Table 17, above). In general, older people should not use drugs like alpha blockers or beta blockers that are prone to causing orthostatic hypotension (a sudden drop in blood pressure upon standing up). These drugs can lead to fainting and falls, a common cause of hip fractures. However, some experts believe that overall health rather than age should be the deciding factor. An otherwise healthy 70-year-old may respond well to medications, while a not-so-healthy 55-year-old may develop side effects.

In sum, know your cardiac risk factors. Monitor your blood pressure regularly. And with lifestyle modifications and medication (if necessary), you should be able to keep blood pressure in a healthy range. ♥

Resources

Organizations

American College of Cardiology
Heart House
2400 N Street NW
Washington DC, 20037
800-253-4636 (toll-free)
www.acc.org

This nonprofit medical society provides consumer-focused information about heart disease and its risk factors through a program called CardioSmart, which features health tracking tools, incentive programs, and mobile resources.

American Heart Association
7272 Greenville Ave.
Dallas, TX 75231
800-242-8721 (toll-free)
www.heart.org

This nonprofit organization publishes pamphlets and booklets on preventing and treating hypertension, all at no charge or for a nominal fee. The organization also operates a consumer hotline to answer general questions on heart health.

National Heart, Lung, and Blood Institute
NHLBI Information Center
P.O. Box 30105
Bethesda, MD 20824
301-592-8573
www.nhlbi.nih.gov

This division of the National Institutes of Health (NIH) supports research, training, and education in the prevention, diagnosis, and treatment of cardiovascular disease. Its website provides a wealth of materials on hypertension, diet, and exercise.

Harvard Special Health Reports

The following Special Health Reports from Harvard Medical School provide more information about some of the topics covered in this report. To order them, go to www.health.harvard.edu or call 877-649-9457 (toll-free).

Diseases of the Heart: A compendium of common heart conditions and the latest treatments
Deepak L. Bhatt, M.D., Medical Editor
(Harvard Medical School, 2016)

This report explains various conditions that affect the heart (including peripheral artery disease, coronary artery disease, heart rhythm disorders, and more) along with their causes, symptoms, diagnosis, and prevention.

The Harvard Medical School 6-Week Plan for Healthy Eating
Teresa Fung, Sc.D., R.D, L.D.N., Medical Editor
Kathy McManus, M.S., R.D., L.D.N., Nutrition Editor
(Harvard Medical School, 2015)

This report will help you analyze your diet, establish goals for healthy meals and snacks, and incorporate practical changes to make your healthy diet a reality. It teaches you how to make just a few dietary changes each week to help you learn a new pattern of healthy eating.

Lose Weight and Keep It Off: Smart approaches to achieving and maintaining a healthy weight
W. Scott Butsch, M.D., M.S.C., Medical Editor
Karen Ansel, M.S., R.D., C.D.N., Nutrition Editor
(Harvard Medical School, 2017)

This report provides step-by-step guidance for weight loss—from selecting a satisfying diet to learning tips and tricks that will help you outwit cravings, sidestep temptation, and control comfort eating. It also includes information on additional lifestyle changes that will help you shed pounds. For those who need further help, there is guidance on weight-loss programs, weight-loss medications, and weight-loss surgery.

Starting to Exercise
Lauren E. Elson, M.D., Medical Editor
Michele Stanten, Fitness Consultant
(Harvard Medical School, 2015)

This report answers many important questions about physical activity, from how exercise changes your body to what diseases it helps prevent. It will also help guide you through starting and maintaining an exercise program that suits your abilities and lifestyle.

Walking for Health: Why this simple form of activity could be your best health insurance
Lauren E. Elson, M.D., Medical Editor
Michele Stanten, Fitness Consultant
(Harvard Medical School, 2015)

You've been walking since you were a toddler, so what could you possibly need to learn? This report introduces you to information on what shoes to wear, safety tips, proper gait, different walking styles, walking for weight loss, and staying motivated.